Dental Health Education

Lesson Planning & Implementation

Lori Gagliardi, RDA, RDH, MEd
Dental Health Educator, Pasadena City College
Department of Life Sciences and Allied Health
Pasadena, California
Cerritos Community College, Department of Health Occupations
Norwalk, California

Appleton & Lange
Stamford, Connecticut

www.appletonlange.com

99 00 01 02 03 / 10 9 8 7 6 5 4 3 2 1

Prentice Hall International (UK) Limited, *London*
Prentice Hall of Australia Pty. Limited, *Sydney*
Prentice Hall Canada, Inc., *Toronto*
Prentice Hall Hispanoamericana, S.A., *Mexico*
Prentice Hall of India Private Limited, *New Delhi*
Prentice Hall of Japan, Inc., *Tokyo*
Simon & Schuster Asia Pte. Ltd., *Singapore*
Editora Prentice Hall do Brasil Ltda., *Rio de Janeiro*
Prentice Hall, *Upper Saddle River, New Jersey*

Library of Congress Cataloging-in-Publication Data

Gagliardi, Lori.
    Dental health education : lesson planning and implementation /
Lori Gagliardi.
        p.   cm.
    ISBN 0-8385-1574-6 (pbk. : alk. paper)
    1. Dental health education.   I. Title.
RK60.8.G34   1998
372.3'7—dc21   98-3597
                                                                CIP

ISSN: 0092-8682

Acquisitions Editor: Kimberly Davies
Production Editor: Mary Ellen McCourt
Art Coordinator: Eve Siegel
Illustrations: Dan Knopsnyder
Interior Designer: Angela Foote
Cover Design: Mary Skudlarek

ISBN 0-8385-1574-6
90000
9 780838 515747

PRINTED IN THE UNITED STATES OF AMERICA

This I Believe

A hundred years from now it
will not matter where I lived,
where *I worked* or where I've been,
but the world may be different
because I was important in
contributing to a child's education.
Teeth that will last a lifetime
begin with early prevention.

—anonymous author with additions by Lori Gagliardi

*This book is dedicated with a heart full
of love and thankfulness to:*

My husband Joe, my sons Anthony and Mark,
and my parents and inlaws—
for their unselfish time
and never-ending support
with my endless projects and commitments,

My friends and colleagues,
for their encouragement,

and

All the professionals dedicated
to helping children prevent dental disease
. . . It begins with education; thus,
the future smiles are in your hands!

Acknowledgments

Special thanks to Pat Stewart, RDH, ED, and Sally McIver, RDH, BS, for the original development of this book as a course syllabus in Dental Health Education. As Sally retired and Pat moved on they graciously gave me their materials and course syllabus with all their blessings. I'm happy to say that after five years of adding my own materials; attending many S.B. 111 workshops, conferences, and training programs, as well as project sharing and contributions from many dental health educators within the S.B. 111, our course syllabus has now become a book.

I would also like to acknowledge all the coordinators and staff from the Children's Dental Disease Prevention Program S.B. 111, Department of Health Services, California, and other programs for their creativity.

Pat Stewart, RDH, ED
Cerritos College
Norwalk, CA

Sally McIver, RDH, BS
Cerritos College (retired)
Norwalk, CA

S.B. 111 Programs
Alameda County Health Care Services, Karen Kopriva, RDH, BS, Jared Fine, DDS, MPH
Contra Costa County Health Department, Lynn Pilant, RDH
Long Beach Department of Health Services, Rosemary Flocken and Barbara Wittington
Los Angeles County Office of Education, Marie Grant
Orange County Health Care Agency, Pauline Geiger, RDH
Sacramento County Dental Program, Kate Varanelli, RDH, MS
San Bernadino Department of Public Health, Arlene Glube, RDH, Carolyn Baker, RDA
San Diego City, Francis Riley, RN, Beverly Hom, RDH
San Diego County Health Department, Kay Stuckardt, RDH, MS
Stanislaus County Health Services, Rose Ann Peterson
Tulare County Department of Health Services, Charlotte Crawford, Fresno County

Additional Programs
Arizona Department of Health Services, Oral Health
California Dental Association, Council on Community Health, Julie Jarrett, RDA
The Dental Health Foundation and the Department of Health Services, Sacramento, Andrea Azevedo, BDS, MPH, Joann Wellman-Benson, RDH, MPH, Mary Maurer, M.ED, and Robert Isman, DDS, MPH
University of Southern California, Diane Melrose, RDH, BS
University of the Pacific (UOP), Janet Chan Fricke, CDA, RDA

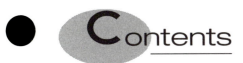

Contents

	Introduction	xi
ʃectioN oNe	**Before You Begin**	**1**
	Community Dental Health Education	3
	Multicultural Issues in Dental Health	7
	Teaching Methods	9
	Classroom Presentation	13
	Classroom Management	17
ʃectioN two	**Planning and Implementing a Dental Health Lesson Plan**	**19**
	The Use of Fluoride	27
	The Importance of Plaque Control	39
	Toothbrushing for Good Oral Health	49
	Flossing for Good Oral Health	59
	Nutrition and Healthy Teeth	67
	Dental Safety and Oral Injury Prevention	79
	Anti-tobacco Lessons	89
	The Dental Office Visit	105
	Last Visit; Wrap Up and Review	121
	Children With Special Needs	135
ʃectioN tHree	**Creating a Community Outreach Program**	**145**
	Dental Health Fair	147
	Parent Education Meeting	153
ʃectioN ſour	**Integrating Dental Health Education into the Classroom**	**168**
	Hints to Help Integrate the Dental Program Into the Academic Curriculum	169
	Visual Aids	173
	Appendix: Additional Resources	*183*
	Recommended Dental Titles	205
	Glossary	*207*
	Bibliography	*209*

Introduction

Dental disease is the most widespread public health problem among the school-age population in the United States today. In some states, 95 percent of children have dental disease in the form of dental caries and gingivitis. Dental disease in a child can and does result in significant lifetime dental disability, dental pain, bleeding gums, missing teeth, time lost from school and work, and the need for dentures. Poor nutrition can also be a contributing factor. The cost of treating the results of dental disease is close to $4.5 billion per year in some states.*

Dental disease in children and the resultant abnormalities in adults can be prevented by education and treatment programs, beginning at an early age. Community dental disease prevention programs can be established for schoolchildren in kindergarten through sixth grade and in classes for children with special needs by local dental health professionals, volunteers, and students in the health care professions. Educational programs should focus on the development of personal practices by students that promote dental health and self awareness. Topics to be emphasized would include causes and prevention of dental diseases, nutrition, dental health and safety, and the need for regular visits to the dental office. The goals of a dental disease prevention program in the classroom are to:

- Instill self-awareness and responsibilities in dental health.
- Encourage decision making about dental health issues.
- Enable students to develop appropriate skills to prevent dental disease.
- Instill positive values and attitudes about dental health to ensure lifelong learning.

A comprehensive dental health program in the classroom is based on the concept of the "whole child," in which dental health is viewed as an integral part of total body health. Through this approach, it is hoped that learning about dental health will be integrated as part of students' school-based education rather than being merely a fragmented portion of classroom instruction.

To meet the goals described above, classroom lessons presented in an organized manner have proven to be the most effective approach. Learning good habits requires a change in behavior. Constant practice, repetition, and reinforcement are necessary. The information given must be the same for every child, otherwise the result will be merely confusion; no learning will take place. Changing students' oral hygiene habits, values, and attitudes toward dental health is the best—as well as the most cost-effective—way to solve dental health problems among the school-age population.

A typical dental disease prevention program would include:

- An initial needs assessment survey (done by the school nurse, volunteer dentist, or hygienists)
- In-service training to the participating classroom teachers, staff, nurse, and any others involved

*S.B. 111, California Department of Health Services, 1996.

- Dental health presentations to the classroom throughout the school year, integrating this information into the regular curriculum as much as possible
- Parent involvement through parent–teacher association (PTA), advisory groups, newsletters, and newspaper articles providing publicity on the program
- Supplies (toothbrushes and floss) for the students to use in dry brushing and flossing the teeth daily under the supervision of the classroom teacher

This text consists of four sections. Section One addresses the roles of the dental health educator and issues you should be aware of before planning and implementing your presentations. Before you begin, keep in mind that it is the responsibility of the dental health educator to be aware of the various factors that influence learning and behavioral change: The learning level of the targeted students, classroom environment, cultural factors, language barriers, amount of time available, and so forth. These are some of the factors you will need to address before entering the classroom. The more knowledgeable you are about the specific group to whom you are presenting, the better able you will be to deliver an effective presentation.

Section Two presents the actual content of the dental health education program. In this text, dental health topics are broken up into lesson plans covering eight essential areas of dental health education:

- The use of fluoride
- The importance of plaque control
- Toothbrushing for plaque control
- Flossing for good oral health
- Nutrition and healthy teeth
- Dental safety and oral injury prevention
- The use of anti-tobacco products
- The dental office visit

Also included in Section Two is information on targeting a special needs classroom.

The lesson plans are organized using Hunter's (1977) five-step lesson plan, modified to include a preparation segment at the beginning and a time frame to keep you on track. The following format is used throughout this text:

- Preparation (things to do before beginning the lesson)
- Anticipatory planning (introduction of the lesson and materials needed)
- General objectives (what students will gain from the lesson)
- Instruction/information (the bulk of the lesson that is new and exciting for students)
- Guided practice activities (to reinforce the information taught)
- Closure (restatement of the objectives to test knowledge)

Presentation of each lesson should take approximately 30 minutes. All of the information for presenting a lesson, suggested activities, and individual lesson plan outline are included for each topic. It will be up to the reader to determine the students' current learning level, and what goals and objectives are obtainable. Therefore, information from the objectives (at the corresponding grade level) may be added to or deleted as needed. Lesson plans and information (e.g., plaque control and brushing) may also be combined into one lesson. However, I would caution against combining more than two topics in any one lesson plan.

Section Three describes the components of a community outreach program and provides two sample programs. The community outreach program is designed to encourage parent involvement in the child's dental health and school-ing. We know parent participation is a vital link to achieving healthy teeth that can last a lifetime. Exhaustive research has proven that parents can make a signif-icant difference in their children's achievement at all age levels. For students, the positive outcome of effective school–family collaboration include: Higher grades and test scores, better attendance, fewer special education placements, and more positive attitudes. Parents are the primary educators of young children, and parental example is the most effective method of establishing positive oral health habits in children.

Section Four emphasizes approaches for integrating dental health into the reg-ular academic curriculum, and the development of visual aids to assist you in your presentations. This section provides suggestions to help you keep dental health education alive in the classroom throughout the year and to prevent frag-mented learning. The goal is to ensure that dental health is not only addressed when dental health educators are present. A list of recommended dental titles concludes this section.

Section Four is followed by an appendix of additional resources and a glos-sary. The appendix provides additional resources: The California Dental Associa-tion's fact sheets on dental care, tooth-talking vocabulary words, and a listing of additional dental health educational resources.

In conclusion, I would like to acknowledge that this text uses many of the les-son plans developed by many educators participating in California's S.B. 111 Children's Dental Disease Prevention Program and many other prevention pro-grams throughout the nation. Many people have contributed their ideas, knowl-edge, and time toward ensuring the success of dental health education in the classroom. Although these individuals may not be recognized by name, their ex-pertise in planning and implementing dental health programs deserves to be noted.

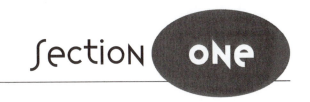
Before You Begin

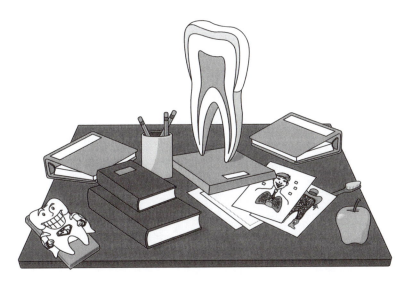

This section covers the roles of the dental hygienist or the dental health educator in community dental health education and discusses issues you should be aware of before planning and implementing your presentation. As I emphasized in the introduction, before you begin, you should review factors that influence intrinsic behavior changes, multicultural issues, teaching methods, emotional and physical development of children in grades K through 6, classroom presentation, and classroom management. Remember that the more knowledge you have about the specific group to whom you will be presenting, the better able you will be to deliver an effective message.

Community Dental Health Education

Many dental hygiene students picture themselves after graduation working for a general dentist or a periodontist as the preventive dental health specialist providing services for several patients each day. However, at some point in your career, you may wish to add a little variety to the daily office routine.

Dental hygienists were originally thought of and trained as oral health educators. Over the years, hygienists have been utilized in this capacity by working in settings such as schools, hospitals, nursing homes, general industry, public health facilities, and so on. Although in any of these settings hygienists may spend some time performing preventive services, the majority of their time probably is spent in education and administration.

It was common in the 1950s and 1960s to encounter dental hygienists who were employed part-time or full-time by local school districts. Often, a mobile "dental trailer" was set up at a school where children received dental health instruction and were screened for dental decay. Local dentists then followed up with either free or low-cost dental care for the needy. As federal funding dwindled, however, these positions were eliminated for the most part in the western United States. The eastern states were more fortunate; local funding and support there have enabled many local dental health programs, coordinated by salaried dental hygienists, to continue their operations with additional dental hygiene preventive services.

Today, dental health is receiving a higher priority at the national level, and more state funds are being allocated for local dental health programs. Elementary schools have been targeted for the 1990s and into the future to meet the *Healthy People 2000* objective of decreasing dental disease among U.S. children.

Community involvement is an essential aspect of a professional career. Now is the time to become involved in the future by educating children in ways to prevent and eliminate dental disease. You can play a vital role as an educator in community dental health programs wherever you live.

Before becoming an active participant in a dental health program, you will need to become familiar with the issues that are discussed on the following pages.

What Is a Comprehensive Dental Health Program?

A comprehensive dental health program is based on the concept of teaching the "whole child," emphasizing dental health as an integral part of total body health. Through this approach, it is hoped that learning about dental health will not be merely a fragmented portion of instruction but instead will be integrated throughout the child's education.

Why Attempt Such a Comprehensive, Time-consuming Program?

In the past few years, the dental community has expressed an increasing interest in school dental health. However, because of a lack of funding, most involvement has been on a volunteer basis. Typically, a dentist or dental hygienist wishing to serve the community has volunteered to visit from one to many classrooms during the course of a school year. In such nonpaying programs, the participants' time commitment was often minimal, so classroom instruction was usually given as a "one-shot" presentation to as many children as possible. No matter how good the intentions of these volunteers, this type of instruction has been proven to be ineffective for several reasons:

- Constant practice, repetition, and reinforcement is necessary. Learning good oral hygiene habits requires a change in behavior. For instance, daily brushing and flossing have been shown to have a positive effect on dental health.
- The information given must be the same for every child. Otherwise, the result will be merely confusion; no learning will take place. Children often receive misinformation about dental health at home, so consistency at school is of the utmost importance.
- Any effective program needs to coordinate scheduling, supplies, evaluations, and so on. Volunteers generally do not have the time to take on these tasks.
- Follow-up referrals for emergency and preventive services are needed. Because of financial considerations, most dentists today are simply unable to render services to all needy families at a reduced cost. This service is usually provided by dental clinics, if, that is, parents have the necessary transportation and finances to utilize these services—and recognize the importance of seeking needed dental care.

Table 1–1 Factors That Influence Intrinsic Behaviors

Knowledge	Statistics show that only about 40% of the population visit the dentist in any one year, many of those only for relief of pain. It would seem that lack of knowledge is the most logical reason for the majority of the population not seeking preventive dental care. However, this is not the case. Today, as we teach dental health concepts to either individual patients or groups, many other factors must be taken into consideration. Some variables include social, cultural, economic, and demographic attributes. A false assumption is that increasing a person's dental health knowledge will help change dental behavior.
Attitudes	This refers to the reactions of an individual to the learning he or she acquires. Attitudes develop slowly through a continuum of low-level experiences or suddenly, from one intense experience. Learned behavior stems from attitudes.
Values	Values usually refer to what a person feels is right or should be done. Every individual establishes a priority of value based on past experiences, which will influence his or her behavior. Even young children may demonstrate attitudes and values developed by modeling parents and teachers. Further, behavior change may take a lot longer for one child than another. Health educators also have attitudes and values that influence their behavior and the aspects of health instruction they emphasize. An educator must consider his or her own points of view relative to health and education. What do you value in relation to dental health and dental health education?
Motivation	The process of motivation involves the following steps: • A specific need • Action/behavior by the individual • A goal to be achieved • Some form of satisfaction If any step in this process is missing, frustration will replace motivation.

Who Is Involved in a Comprehensive Dental Health Program?

The following persons will need to be involved in your program:

- Superintendent of schools
- Principal
- Health services coordinator
- School nurse
- Classroom teacher
- Local dental, dental hygiene, and dental assistants
- PTA/School support groups

Changing students' oral hygiene habits is the best way to solve the public health problem of dental disease among the school-age population. However, changing these habits involves factors that are intrinsic to behavioral change: knowledge, attitudes, values, and motivation. Table 1–1 can help you identify your own intrinsic behaviors. Once you have established your own intrinsic behaviors, use this table to assess how you will create behavioral changes within the population for whom you will be providing dental health education.

Multicultural Issues in Dental Health

Educators in today's classrooms are presented with a tremendously diverse student population. According to the Los Angeles County Office of Education, 90 languages are spoken in just that one area of the state. Each of these languages represents cultural as well as language barriers when it comes to communicating a dental health lesson in the classroom. Dental health educators must be sensitive to the needs of the ever-growing diversity of cultural backgrounds present in the classroom.

Communication and cultural diversity are closely interwoven. Communication, as defined by *Merriam-Webster's Collegiate Dictionary* (1993), refers to "a process by which information is exchanged between individuals through a common system of symbols, signs, or behavior." Culture is defined as "the customary beliefs, social norms, and material traits of a racial, religious, or social group." For many students, the information on dental health that is presented in the classroom may be very different from the culturally influenced teaching they have received within their family or community.

It can be said that most cultures have five major components:

1. A pattern of communication
2. A basic diet
3. A common style of dress
4. Common socialization patterns
5. A common set of values and beliefs

Cultural diversity influences how individuals express themselves, both verbally and nonverbally. Cultural patterns are embedded beginning at birth in child-rearing practices. The communication practices of individual cultures affect the expression of ideas, feelings, and decision making. Variations in communication practices may be widespread (e.g., common to an entire cultural group), or limited to the use of particular words or gestures with specific meanings for a small group (e.g., the family). In addition, within a given culture is a set of values and beliefs that guide members' social communication.

What is accepted in one culture may be entirely inappropriate in another. For instance, Anglo-Americans may be more likely to conceal feelings than persons from other cultural groups, and the United States in general is considered a low-touch culture. In comparison, a member of a Middle-Eastern or Mediterranean culture may be open and loud with expressions, and rely on touch as an important part of communication. Similarly, the dominant American cultural values emphasize competition and individual achievement whereas many other cultures emphasize cooperation and group achievement.

The following example illustrates how this information can be applied to dental health education. Suppose you wanted to test the knowledge of a group of students. You might choose to question the students individually. But again, suppose that their cultural background is one that emphasizes group achievement. In this instance, the classroom response to the dental health lesson would probably be very low. The educator must always remember that a dental health program that has been presented successfully to one class or group may have to be modified to fit another group. Cultural characteristics, language barriers, and a preference for cooperative rather than individual learning will all influence the educator's task. Thus, the educator should attempt to adapt the content and teaching approach of the lesson to meet the needs of the particular group of students.

Finally, remember that although all of us are influenced by our cultures, we remain individuals. It is difficult to accurately describe the characteristics of any cultural group, particularly as each new generation has an influence on its culture. When the dental health educator is sensitive to all cultures that may be represented in the classroom, he or she will be most effective in presenting information that can be absorbed by all students.

t eaching Methods

Many different strategies can be used in teaching, among them: lecture, demonstration, discussion, inquiry, games, and activities. Not all can be handled effectively by everyone. Practice at least three of the methods that follow to determine which ones best fit your style and personality. As always, be sure the information presented is appropriate to the cognitive and physical level of the students, as outlined in Table 1–2.

Lecture

The most traditional teaching method, lecture, is probably the easiest for the Dental Health Educator—who need simply develop material, memorize it, and deliver it verbatim to the class. Unfortunately, learning does not always follow at the level expected. This failure to meet educational goals may stem from:

- A monotone style of presentation that fails to hold listeners' attention.
- A learning experience that is passive rather than active.
- A format that does not lend itself to questions or feedback.

Among educators today, there is a tendency to depart from the traditional lecture format by using a different approach entirely or combining this method with one or two others.

Demonstration

As a teaching method, demonstration can be an effective tool, especially if the students' interest has been previously stimulated. Most often this method is combined with lecture, which has the advantage of involving two senses (hearing and seeing) instead of just one. Problems associated with demonstration include:

- Materials that are too cumbersome to carry with you
- For large groups, the need for special facilities so that everyone can see the demonstration
- Inability for one person to do the demonstration alone

When teaching about dental health, demonstration becomes a key element in each presentation. You will want to perfect this method before focusing on others. Audiovisual aids fit into this category.

Discussion

Control of the class is a major determinant of success or failure when employing discussion. This teaching method is usually most effective in small groups. An introductory lecture, demonstration, research assignment, or group sharing of dental experiences may be needed to stimulate students' interest and prepare them for this activity.

Inquiry

Inquiry—the technique of asking questions to stimulate learning—is probably the most effective teaching method. However, it requires a considerable amount of skill on the part of the teacher. With this teaching method, the class is expected to

Table 1–2   Emotional and Physical Development of Children

Age/Grade	Emotional Characteristics	Physical Characteristics
5/Kindergarten	Very direct Very interested in health problems and "why" Enjoys talking Personal Realistic Accepts help Basically kind	Skips, hops Laces shoes Fastens buttons Likes to copy Holds a toothbrush Swishes without swallowing
6/First grade	Explores everything Easily distracted Changes activity easily Wants to succeed Wants to obey rules Demanding and stubborn	Awkward in fine motor tasks Much oral activity: blows, bites lips, chews pencils Takes things apart Ties shoes Copies more accurately
7/Second grade	Wants to be perfect Hoards time and attention Sensitive feelings Less distracted Poor loser	Enjoys pencils, drawing, writing Balances better Personal care is better: dresses easily, brushes hair and teeth
8/Third grade	Curious Listens and watches More conscious of relationships Curious about body, what causes disease, nature, what cures More dramatic Likes clubs, rules Interests are short-lived Argues Needs help in care of possessions Likes riddles	Very active Faster and smoother in finer motor activities More graceful Can ride a bike More social Manipulative skills improve
9/Fourth grade	Self-motivated Does not enjoy routine tasks Interested in perfecting skills Better able to perform self-appraisal Can accept criticism and fairness Reasonable Responsible Awed by self, own ideas, power and body	Difficult to calm after an activity More energy
10/Fifth grade	Has heroes, loyalties, interest in social justice Likes secret clubs Interested in body and how it works Little concern about personal grooming and health	Enjoys team sports Interested in exercising Wants big muscles
11/Sixth grade	Self-conscious about body and how it appears to others Interest in body differences Focus on personal health, grooming, and being in style	Exercise is important

achieve the highest level of learning through self-discovery and reflection. A major concept is that the learner is exposed to a certain degree of frustration, which stimulates the thinking process more than rote memorization.

Little information or direction is given initially. The teacher asks questions to help the learner solve his or her own problems. For example, a dental health educator who wishes to teach an elementary school class what teeth are used for might ask a series of questions, such as:

1. "Why do you suppose we have teeth?" This first question will probably elicit some correct answers, but usually not all possibilities.
2. "Can you think of any other reasons we have teeth?" At this point, the educator must allow ample time for the students to think through the question and produce additional answers.

If the educator had begun by saying, "We have teeth for several reasons. Teeth help us chew our food, smile, talk, and so on," the children would be given some points to memorize. More than likely they would be unable to remember all the answers a short time later. By using the inquiry method, however, the children are compelled to think about how they use their own teeth and then come up with the answers. Children who learn in this way are much more likely to remember the lesson.

Games and Activities

If handled properly, games and activities can be incorporated into any of the previously mentioned teaching methods. To be successful, however, they must be well planned and organized with an objective in mind. This method is one of the best ways to stimulate interest and participation in the elementary school classroom.

Classroom Presentation

There are several aspects of classroom presentation that you will need to address before becoming an effective educator. These aspects may come naturally to you, or some or all aspects may be intermittently or continually frustrating. However, your efforts to master these aspects will improve your presentations.

Initial Fear of Speaking in Front of an Audience

It is perfectly normal to be nervous or, in some cases, terrified when facing an audience. The best way to control this anxiety is to be well prepared for your presentation. Here are a few tips:

- Do not rely on reading notes.
- Do not rely on your partner to take over.
- Do prepare in front of an audience—this will help you feel comfortable and may also provide you with feedback on your speaking voice, level of enthusiasm, and body language.
- Do speak up! If you speak with assurance, the quiver in your voice will shortly disappear.
- Practice!
- Anticipate problems. Nothing is more unnerving than to plan to introduce a film only to find that the projector is broken or unavailable. Always rehearse an alternative plan and be sure additional equipment, if needed, is requested in advance.
- Encourage questions from your audience. Their participation will allow you a moment to relax and let your heart stop pounding.

Initially, your presentations may be limited for the most part to a lecture that simply introduces facts. Once you begin to relax in front of the classroom, however, you can begin to think about other aspects of your presentation, such as audiovisual aids and interactive components.

Quality of Audiovisual Aids, Demonstration, and/or Participation Techniques

When developing audiovisual aids or other interactive strategies for your presentation, keep the following points in mind:

- Do make sure everyone can see the demonstration, poster, or other display. Hold it up long enough for the children to read or interpret the message.
- Walk around the classroom if necessary so that everyone can see.
- If you pass out materials, make sure everyone has a chance to see, hold, or feel the item before you move on to the next step.
- Try to establish eye contact with everyone in the room.
- Do not demonstrate toothbrushing, flossing, or other techniques on yourself while trying to give directions verbally.
- Make sure all children begin a procedure together.

- Giving directions for a group procedure requires some thought. Be sure directions are clear and concise. You may need to repeat directions several times in the elementary school classroom.
- Be sure you have thoroughly demonstrated the expected behavior (i.e., holding the toothbrush properly and brushing in a sequence) before passing out supplies. This will ensure that the attention of the audience will be focused on you.

Teaching Concepts

Once your presentation is well under control, you will be able to scrutinize your message and the effectiveness of the communication. This would include:

- Being aware of classroom clues to noncommunication (such as talking, shuffling, looking around the room).
- Summarizing difficult concepts through demonstration, interpretive question and answer, class discussion, and so on.
- Obtaining the anticipated answer to your questions, rather than simply a "yes" or "no" response.
- Observing problems in brushing and flossing technique and correcting them immediately.
- Being an active listener and beginning to answer questions spontaneously in more detail. At this point, some questions may allow you to explain a new concept without having to rely on a prepared script.
- Being aware of items in the classroom than can enhance your presentation. Oftentimes, teachers display projects related to dental health. These related materials provide an opportunity to: (1) compliment the class and/or teacher, thus establishing rapport; (2) reinforce a concept already introduced; and (3) introduce a new concept by building on one already introduced.

Motivation Through Feelings

This aspect involves affective learning; helping the class to express their feelings and attitudes, and perhaps reflect on or establish values related to dental health. Achieving this goal is difficult, particularly with younger elementary school children. Techniques to accomplish this would include:

- Role playing
- Structured values activities
- Learning games
- Small group interaction

Most of the activities throughout this book are geared toward motivating the class through experiences and feelings. Don't be afraid to be creative. Keep in mind, however, that the concepts you are teaching should remain consistent and appropriate for the grade level or the particular classroom. If you have good ideas and you feel the lesson was successful, by all means share it!

An Eight-step Model for Planning Instruction

After reviewing the preceding information, you should have a good idea of the specific techniques you want to use in your presentation to a targeted group. Now you need to put your lesson plan together. You can begin by utilizing the eight-step planning model developed by Renner (1985). This model will also be used to incorporate more specific information that applies to Hunter's (1971) five-step lesson plan, which is presented in Section Two.

Determine Objectives

The easiest place to begin is to write down your goals and objectives for each presentation. Determine what you expect your students to be able to do and know by the end of the lesson and how you would like them to think and feel. Be specific with your objectives. Avoid generalities such as "the student will appreciate the value of good dental health." If your objectives are measurable, it will be easier to assess whether they have been met at the end of the presentation.

Access Your Own Skills

By now you have an idea of what works for you—your teaching style. Plan your program around your personality, your attitudes, your knowledge, and your interests. Play on your individual strengths.

Determine the Learners' Skill

Seek out those who can give you insight (teachers) into the needs and abilities of your prospective learners (students). Conference with the group contact person. Arrange a visit purely for observation. Talk to colleagues who have worked with this or a similar group in the past. The better prepared you are—the easier it will be to plan and present information that is of value to your audience. They will appreciate the fact that you did your homework and are able to relate to their specific level and needs.

Survey the System

The school, company, staff, institution, or other setting in which your program will take place often influences who attends, what is expected, and what is likely to happen. Discover any rules that may affect your presentation and any administrative constraints that may apply. Note the atmosphere of the facility (relaxed, stiff, formal, academic, happy, liberal, etc.).

Choose Appropriate Teaching/Learning Strategies

Certain strategies are more suitable for certain learning objectives. In general, a combination of demonstrations, lectures, and plenty of practice yield desired results. Read the section on classroom presentation and determine what will work best for your group based on their needs, motivation, and abilities.

Utilize Outside Resources

Plan ahead by listing films, slides, handouts, supplies (e.g., toothbrushes, floss), and any audiovisuals and other items that might enhance your presentation. Remember that supplies have to be ordered and films reserved and all of this takes time.

Incorporate Evaluation and Feedback

Build into your presentation opportunities for frequent feedback, keeping in mind that when you complete your self-evaluation or receive the evaluation from the contact person in a community outreach program, it will not be too late to change or improve your presentation. Solicit feedback often throughout your presentations by asking questions such as the following:

- "Before I go on, does this make sense to you?"
- "Am I going too fast?"
- "Did I lose you?"
- "Are there any questions you want me to answer?"
- "You seem confused" (responding to nonverbal signs), "can I help?"

Try not to answer your own questions too often. Devise questions based on information and knowledge, making it difficult for students to answer with a simple "yes" or "no" response.

Provide for Restructuring

Allow for flexibility and change by keeping your outline (lesson plan) brief and your ideas "pencilled in." Remember that your presentation is a proposed outline, only. It may have to be changed as you become more familiar with your participants' abilities and needs.

Additional Presentation Techniques

Here are a few final tips that you can use to improve your presentations:

- Be sure to start your presentation on time and be prepared. When working with a partner, don't wait until you are in front of the classroom to decide who is going to talk first. Don't begin your lesson by fumbling around for a visual aid.
- Don't begin the lesson until the class has settled down and is ready to pay attention to you.
- Make sure the students can actually read before asking them to do so.
- Choose an appropriate vocabulary. Younger children may be confused by words such as "tissues," "maintain," "promote," and so on.
- When passing items around the room for visual inspection, stop the lesson until the items have all been returned to you; otherwise you will lose your audience.
- Similarly, when resuming your lecture after an activity such as playing a game or coloring a handout, tell the children to put away these materials before continuing with the lesson.
- Plan to use the blackboard whenever possible. Be sure to print or write using letters that match those the children are being taught, and write large enough so that all the students can read what you have written.
- Call on a variety of children. There will always be one or two who will raise their hands before you have even finished asking a question. Try waiting a bit longer, then say, "Let's give someone else [or another group/table] a chance."
- One of the most important elements in successful learning is making sure all the children can hear what is being said. In most classes, a child's question will not be heard by any of the children sitting behind him or her. Always repeat the question before beginning your answer. This also provides a chance to clarify or expand on the question.
- *Listen carefully to questions.* Oftentimes, questions give you a great opportunity to discuss or clarify an important concept. Remember, if one child asks the question, many others may be thinking the same thing.
- Don't be surprised if you find you need to repeat directions several times during a session of brushing or flossing or other activities.

Classroom Management

Research has shown that students perform better academically when teachers are good classroom managers. Students in these situations learn and retain more than students of teachers who are not good classroom managers.

Teachers who are good classroom managers share the following traits. They:

- Are clear about their expectations and clearly present directions, objectives, and the purpose of the lesson.
- Present information in small steps.
- Allow students to practice.
- Monitor and provide feedback.
- Plan ahead by being prepared, establishing signals, taking charge, rewarding task-oriented behaviors, being positive, being specific, and providing immediate reinforcement.

In addition, these teachers:

- Stay calm.
- Deal with problems immediately.
- Have a secure routine.
- Teach at the correct level of difficulty.
- Are enthusiastic.
- Use humor.
- Speak at the right voice level.
- Use appealing visuals, which can be seen by everyone.
- Question and respond appropriately.
- Use a variety of teaching methods that appeal to three types of learners: auditory, visual, and kinesthetic.
- Use active participation techniques such as discussing with a partner, brainstorming, using signals (finger, thumb, eye), encouraging unison responses, including activities appropriate to children's motor development, getting one student to respond (agree or disagree), flashing answers to the group, and using flash cards.

By using these techniques, you can improve your own classroom management skills and enhance your ability to deliver effective dental health presentations to a variety of students.

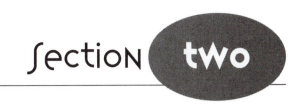

Planning and Implementing a Dental Health Lesson Plan

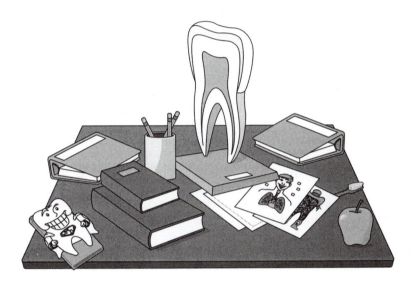

this section begins with an overview of a five-step lesson plan that can be used to present dental health information. As discussed in the introduction to this book, the goals of a dental disease prevention program in the classroom are to:

- Instill self-awareness and responsibilities in dental health.
- Encourage decision making about dental health issues.
- Enable students to develop appropriate skills to prevent dental disease.
- Instill positive values and attitudes about dental health to ensure lifelong learning.

Many aspects of preventive education might be covered in any one particular lesson. In this text, I have targeted specific areas of dental health that can be emphasized at the appropriate grade level. The topics are broken up into lesson plans covering eight essential areas of dental health education, as follows:

- The use of fluoride
- The importance of plaque control
- Toothbrushing for plaque control

- Flossing for good oral health
- Nutrition and healthy teeth
- Dental safety and oral injury prevention
- The use of anti-tobacco products
- The dental office visit

These topics conclude with a final chapter focusing on the last visit (wrap up and review). Also included in this section is information on targeting a special needs classroom of students.

The lesson plans are organized using Hunter's (1971) five-step lesson plan, described below, which has been modified to include a preparation segment at the beginning and a time frame to keep you on track.

Five-step Lesson Plan

The five-step lesson plan can be used when learning or presenting a new idea or skill. Hunter's five steps include:

1. Anticipatory planning (introduction of the lesson and materials needed)
2. Objectives (what the student will gain from this lesson)
3. Instruction/information (the bulk of the lesson that is new and exciting for the student)
4. Guided practice activities (to reinforce the information taught)
5. Closure (restatement of the objectives to test knowledge)

Some, but not all, steps are appropriate in a review lesson, discussion lesson, or inquiry lesson. The lesson plans in this book are all based on the five-step lesson plan, thus giving the reader an easy guideline to follow. All of the lessons, with the exception of the community outreach programs, provide for a 30-minute presentation. As you gain experience, you will be able to develop your own lesson plans. By using the five-step lesson plan outline and making sure your material is appropriate for the particular grade level, you will ensure the success of your dental health lessons. Use the Quick Check Lesson Plan at the end of this discussion to be sure you have addressed all the information in your own lesson plans.

Preparation (5 minutes)

Before beginning the lesson, obtain necessary materials. Allow adequate time to get to the classroom on time. Be at least 5 minutes early to set up for the presentation.

Anticipatory Planning (5 minutes)

Focus the students' attention. Use a stimulus such as a question, problem, interesting fact, visual (toothbrush, model), and so forth. Establish the purpose for the lesson; that is, why it is important and relevant to students.

Objectives (2–3 minutes)

State the learning objectives. These objectives tell students what they will be able to do by the end of the lesson. The objectives should be specific and measurable. Avoid beginning your objectives with words like "know," "understand," and "learn" because it is difficult to measure the outcome of such concepts. Use words like "identify," "demonstrate," "state," and "write."

Instruction/Information (10 minutes)

This segment may be combined with the guided practice segment (10 to 20 minutes) that follows. To plan this content, first determine what information or skills are needed by the students to accomplish the objective(s) stated previously. Information and skills must reflect the appropriate grade level and skills of the students. Keep the following points in mind when presenting information:

1. Your topic
   a. Explain central concepts.
   b. State definitions of key terms.
   c. Identify critical attributes of concepts and skills.
   d. Illustrate concepts with appropriate examples and visuals.
   e. Model the behavior proposed by the objectives (if including the guided practice activity combination).
2. Possible methods of instruction
   a. Lecture
   b. Demonstration
   c. Inquiry
   d. Visual aids
   e. Black/white board
   f. Felt board
   g. Posters
   h. Audiovisuals
   i. Audiocassettes
   j. Drawing paper
   k. Puppets

Table 2–1 summarizes grade- and age-appropriate instructional guidelines for presenting information on the eight dental health topics included in this section.

Guided Practice Activities (10 minutes)

This segment may be combined with the preceding instruction/information segment (20 minutes) dental health educators need to show examples of the desired behavior or correctly performed skill that is expected by the conclusion. First, explain what students are to do. Then, model or show students how to carry out the objective. Examples are very important to make learning vivid and concrete. The amount of modeling and the number of examples that are needed depend on the complexity of the content, grade level and dexterity of the students, and their ability to learn.

Check for understanding by having the students model the skill being proposed. Be sure to give individual help as needed to guide each student through the skill. The beginning stages of learning are critical in determining future successful performance of any activity. Consequently, the students' initial attempts at learning should be carefully guided to ensure that they are accurate and successful. The students need to perform the complete skill, with clarification or recommendations for improvement occurring immediately as it is needed. In this way, you will be assured that students will be able to perform the skill satisfactorily without assistance rather than practicing mistakes. Be sure to:

- Initiate practice activities that are under your direct supervision.
- Provide close monitoring.
- Continue to check for understanding.
- Provide specific and immediate knowledge of results.

Closure (2–3 minutes)

After completing the guided practice segment, you should feel confident that students can correctly perform the skills that have been presented without assistance. Provide a short, final assessment of the activity, checking for knowledge of the material presented, and asking students to restate the objectives in question form. Encourage students to continue the activity at home.

You should make a conscious decision to add or delete steps in lesson design based on the amount of time allotted. Keep in mind the students' level of learning and the length of their attention span.

Table 2–1 Overview of Dental Health Education Subjects for Grades K–6

Kindergarten

Kindergartners have varying levels of coordination. It is best to gear your instruction toward exposing them to the basic concepts. Emphasize mastery of oral hygiene techniques to the greatest degree possible.

Objectives

- Fluoride: Identify that fluoride contributes to oral health.
- Plaque control: Describe plaque; indicate that plaque is not pleasant to look at.
- Toothbrushing: Tell how plaque can be disrupted.
- Flossing: Identify dental floss and its function.
- Nutrition: State that a variety of foods are needed to maintain healthy teeth; choose a variety of good foods for their teeth.
- Safety: Name the safety rules to prevent oral injury.
- Anti-tobacco products: Distinguish between good and bad habits.
- Dental office: Identify the importance of teeth; identify the dental health team members.

1st Grade

Health teaching revolves around the child and the group in which he or she lives; that is, the class.

Objectives

- Fluoride: Describe topical fluoride.
- Plaque control: Relate dental disease process; identify two consequences of plaque and where it hides.
- Toothbrushing: List characteristics of a good toothbrush.
- Flossing: Identify the importance of flossing.
- Nutrition: Identify key food groups and describe pyramid.
- Safety: Explain procedure for knocked-out tooth.
- Anti-tobacco products: List three ways to protect yourself from sidestream smoke.
- Dental office: Explain functions of a dental sealant; describe instruments used in a dental office; identify various duties of the dental health team members.

2nd Grade

Children experience their first accomplishments in school, progressing to the second grade. Dental health is also progressing. The child loses his or her primary teeth and acquires new teeth.

Objectives

- Fluoride: Describe the benefit of using fluoride.
- Plaque control: Describe oral disorders caused by plaque; explain the process of dental disease.
- Toothbrushing: Demonstrate the ability to brush properly.
- Flossing: Demonstrate the ability to hold floss.
- Nutrition: State why certain foods are at the top of the pyramid.
- Safety: Explain the contents and purpose of a dental emergency kit.
- Anti-tobacco products: Identify three body parts affected by tobacco.
- Dental office: Name and describe the functions of teeth.

3rd Grade

Progress in body growth and development leads to an interest in new teeth that are growing, too.

Objectives

- Fluoride: Name and explain the two types of fluoride.
- Plaque control: Identify warning signs of dental disease.
- Toothbrushing: Demonstrate proper grasp and removal of plaque.
- Flossing: Demonstrate the ability to floss.
- Nutrition: Review the pyramid and its importance to dental health.

continues on next page

Table 2–1   Overview of Dental Health Education Subjects for Grades K–6 *continues from previous page*

3rd Grade

- Safety: Describe what to do for various dental emergencies.
- Anti-tobacco products: Recognize that smokeless tobacco is an unsafe alternate to cigarettes and other tobacco products.
- Dental office: Relate the history of dentistry; describe the benefits of modern dentistry.

4th Grade

Interest centers in the functions and care of the body.

Objectives

- Fluoride: Describe fluoride sources.
- Plaque control: Any of the above information.
- Toothbrushing: Discuss signs and causes of periodontal disease.
- Flossing: Any of the above information.
- Nutrition: Any of the above information.
- Safety: Any of the above information.
- Anti-tobacco products: Define peer pressure; list three ways to say "no" to tobacco; list two advertising tricks of tobacco companies.
- Dental office: Any of the above information.

5th Grade

Children have good appetites at this age and interest in food is high. However, they may have little concern about personal health and grooming.

Objectives

- Fluoride: Any of the above information.
- Plaque control: Any of the above information.
- Toothbrushing: Relate the results of dental neglect, decay, and the dental disease process.
- Flossing: Any of the above information.
- Nutrition: Any of the above information.
- Safety: Any of the above information.
- Anti-tobacco products: Any of the above information.
- Dental office: Any of the above information.

6th Grade

Concentration is focused on accident prevention and good health practices. Children at this age are self-conscious about their body and how it appears to others.

Objectives

- Fluoride: Any of the above information.
- Plaque control: Any of the above information.
- Toothbrushing: Any of the above information.
- Flossing: Any of the above information.
- Nutrition: Any of the above information.
- Safety: Any of the above information.
- Anti-tobacco products: Any of the above information.
- Dental office: Careers in dentistry.

Note: The K–6th grade objectives listed here are intended to provide an overall guideline for lesson planning. Keep in mind that students at each grade level may vary as to the dental knowledge and background they have previously been exposed to. Thus, information from any grade level below the level you are planning for should also be incorporated in the lesson. Do not assume that a student at one grade level has mastered all the information that should have been learned prior to that grade level.

Lesson Plan / QUICK CHECK

Anticipatory Planning

_____ Focus students.

_____ Use visuals.

_____ Establish the purpose of the lesson.

_____ Review the previous lesson.

_____ Present an overview of today's goal.

_____ Review classroom rules.

Objectives

_____ State in measureable terms.

Instruction/Information

_____ Provide information.

_____ Explain concepts.

_____ State definitions.

_____ Identify critical attributes.

_____ Provide examples.

_____ Model behaviors or skills.

_____ Use visuals.

_____ Vary teaching methods.

_____ Check for understanding.

Guided Practice Activities

_____ Initiate practice activities.

_____ Provide feedback.

_____ Check for understanding.

Closure

_____ Restate objectives in question form.

_____ Recap today's lesson.

_____ Encourage students to practice the behavior or skill on their own.

_____ Plan next visit.

Additional Comments _____

the Use of Fluoride

Preparation

(5 minutes before beginning lesson)

Bring a variety of items or pictures that contain fluoride, such as green leafy vegetables, fish, or tuna, vitamins, tablets, toothpaste, mouth rinse, water, and gel for fluoride trays. Spell the word "fluoride" on the board. Bring information from your local water department about the addition of fluoride to the public water supply.

Anticipatory Planning

(5 minutes)

- Review the previous lesson, if applicable.
- Introduce presenters.
- Describe the goals of today's lesson, the format of information, or general topics to be covered.
- Review classroom rules (grades K–3), if applicable.
- Survey the classroom's fluoride exposure. (Ask: "How many of you use toothpaste or drink water with fluoride?")

General Objectives by Grade Level

State specifically no more than three objectives appropriate for the classroom learning level that indicate what the majority of the students will be able to achieve by the completion of the lesson. Keep in mind for every grade level you advance, the previous grade level objectives could also be used.

(2–3 minutes)

Upon completion of this lesson, the student will be able to:

GR	OBJECTIVES
K	Identify that fluoride contributes to oral health.
1	Describe topical fluoride.
2	Describe the benefits of using fluoride.
3	Name and explain the two types of fluoride (topical and systemic).
4	Describe fluoride sources.
5	Include any or all of the above information.
6	Include any or all of the above information.

Instruction/Information

(10 minutes)

More than one topic may be included or combined with the guided practice segment (10 to 15 minutes). Use as many visual aids as possible for grades K–3; group discussion may be more appropriate for grades 4–6.

- Review the general information; make a chart comparing the two types of fluoride (topical and systemic).
- Emphasize how fluoride contributes to oral health. (Fluoride is a nutrient and a mineral that makes teeth stronger.)
- Utilize discussion: A happy smile begins with fluoridation.
- Present the history of fluoride.

General information

Fluoride is an essential nutrient necessary for proper bone and tooth formation. It is found in trace amounts in most foods and in varying amounts in water. The most effective and inexpensive way to reduce dental decay in a community is through water fluoridation. Because many areas do not have optimal fluoride levels in the water (approximately 1 part per million), the supplemental use of fluorides has proven extremely effective in the reduction of decay.

A fluoride that is swallowed is called a *systemic fluoride*. It is incorporated into the tooth structure from inside the body. The fluoride ion combines with tooth enamel to make a more perfect crystal (hydroxyapatite, H-5 dental enamel) that is more resistant to decay. Examples of systemic fluorides include fluoridation of city water, fluoride tablets or drops, and very small amounts of fluoride found in foods such as dark green leafy vegetables, fish, and apples.

Fluorides that are exposed directly to the tooth are called *topical fluorides*. Topical fluorides are applied to a tooth after the tooth has erupted into the mouth. Examples of topical fluorides include fluoride toothpaste, mouth rinse, and treatments given by a dentist or dental hygienists or in school fluoride rinse programs.

Fluoride is not the only thing necessary for good dental health, but the protection fluoride gives has been shown to reduce decay from 20 percent to 60 percent, depending on the source, timing, and duration of the fluoride supplement. Fluoride protection in combination with effective plaque removal beginning at an early age and a reduced intake of sweets can contribute to a marked decrease in dental disease for an entire lifetime.

The most effective and inexpensive way to reduce dental decay in a community is through water fluoridation. When this is not utilized, self-applied fluorides are also effective in reducing decay at a minimal cost. A prescription for 0.2 percent sodium fluoride mouth rinse or 0.25 mg tablet benefits children who do not obtain optimal levels of systemic fluoride. (Refer to Tables 2–2 and 2–3 for listings of several different types of fluoride rinses.) Sodium fluoride mouth rinse has been demonstrated to have several advantages when used in a school-based rinsing program; among them: (1) it takes little time (3 to 5 minutes a week), (2) it is inexpensive and simple to distribute to the participants, and (3) its use requires limited professional supervision.

Discussion: A happy smile begins with fluoridation

Topic: Local Water Fluoridation

Visit your local water company. Gather pamphlets, booklets, and other materials pertaining to fluoridation and the water system. Find out how much fluoride is in the local water supply. Is the fluoride natural (from ground water) or added? This lesson is a great way to infuse a dental concept into a science/environment curriculum.

Topic: Body Systems and Water

Our bodies are made up of 70 percent water. Therefore, every system in our body uses water. Review the following questions:

- Why is water important to our teeth?
- What body system does our teeth belong to?

Topic: Minerals in Water

Water is a solvent. Therefore, many minerals are found in water. Review the following questions:

Table 2–2   Fluoride Products for Home Use[a]

Fluoride Rinses, Nonprescription (OTC)

Alcohol Content (6%–12%)
  Fluorigard Anti-cavity Fluoride Rinse (Colgate)   0.05% NaF
  NaFRINSE Neutral Rinse (Colgate)   0.05% NaF
  NaFRINSE Acidulated Oral Rinse (Colgate)   0.05% APF
  Phos Flur Daily Oral Rinse (Colgate)   0.044% APF
Alcohol Free
  Oral-B Rinse Therapy Anti-cavity Treatment (Oral-B)   0.05% NaF
  Reach Act for Kids Fluoride Anti-Cavity (J & J)   0.05% NaF

Directions: 1×/day—1 minute
              Don't eat or drink for 30 minutes

Fluoride Gels, Nonprescription (0.4% SnF$_2$)

  Activus (Colgate)
  Alpha-Dent (Alphadental)
  Easy-Gel (Du-More)
  Gel-Kam (Colgate)
  Gel-Tin (Young)
  Perfect Choice (Challenge Products)
  Plak Smacker (Plak Smacker)
  Pro-Dentx (Pro-Dentec)
  Schein Home Care (Henry Schein)
  Super-Dent (Carlisle Laboratories)

Directions: 1–2×/day—Brush 1 minute; swish 1 minute
              Don't eat or drink for 30 minutes

Fluoride Rinses, Prescription

  NaFRINSE Weekly Rinse (Orachem)   0.2% NaF
  Prevident Dental Rinse (Colgate)   0.2% NaF
  Pro-Dentx Neutral Rinse (Pro-Dentec)   0.2% NaF

Directions: 1×/day OR 1x/week—1 minute
              Don't eat or drink for 30 minutes

Fluoride Drops, Prescription

  Karigel-N (Young Dental)   1.1% NaF
  Thera-Flur-N (Colgate)   1.1% NaF
  Thera-Flur (Colgate)   1.1% APF

Directions: Place drops in a custom form tray.
              1×/day—5 minutes

NaF = sodium fluoride; OTC = over-the-counter products; SnF$_2$ = stannous fluoride; APF = acidulated phosphate fluoride.
[a]These products carry the American Dental Association (ADA) Seal of Acceptance.

- What are the two minerals found in water that are important to our teeth and bones? (*Answer:* Fluoride and calcium.)
- Drinking water can be a good source of fluoride. Is your city water fluoridated?
- How much fluoride should you have in your drinking water to prevent tooth decay (cavities)? (*Answer:* Dentists, doctors, and scientists recommend 1 part per million [ppm]. If you live where the weather is warmer, the recommended amount may be slightly less but never less than 0.7 ppm. This is because in warmer climates, people tend to drink more water. One ppm would be equal to one drop of fluoride in 10 gallons of water.)

Table 2–3   Additional Fluoride Products

Fluoride Gels, Prescription (1.1% NaF)[a]

Perfect Choice Brush-On (Biotrol)
Neutracare (Oral B)
Prevident (Colgate)
Pro-Dentx (Pro-Dentec)

Directions: 1×/day—Brush 1 minute; swish 1 minute
May rinse with water (optional)

Perio Rinses, Prescription (0.63% SnF$_2$—when diluted, 0.01% SnF)

Perfect Choice Perio Rinse (Biotrol)
Periocheck Oral Med (Pro-Dentec)

Directions: Dilute with water (follow instructions)
Rinse 1×/day—1–2 minutes
Don't eat or drink for 30 minutes
May also be used with an oral irrigator

Office Fluorides

ADA Accepted for use with trays or rinse (professional treatment)
    1.23% APF—gel, foam
    2% NaF—gel, foam
    8% SnF$_2$—solution

Directions: 1×/3–6 months—4 minutes

Office Irrigation
    2% NaF
    3.28% SnF$_2$—dilutes to 1.64% SnF$_2$

Office Desensitizers
    33⅓% NaF
    0.171% Desensitizer (contains stannous and acidulated phophate)

APF = acidulated phosphate fluoride; NaF = sodium fluoride; SnF = neutral stannous fluoride; SnF$_2$ = stannous fluoride.
[a]These products are not accepted by the American Dental Association (ADA).

Topic: How Much Fluoride Do We Need?

The water from the utilities must be safe for everyone to use. Fluoride is a naturally occurring mineral found in or added to water. Fluoridation has been studied for almost 50 years and has been found to be safe. Fluoride in the drinking water is one of the most cost-effective ways to reduce dental decay. However, just like

Table 2–4   Systemic Fluoride: Supplemental Fluoride Dosage Schedule (mg/day), 1994

Age	Domestic Water Fluoride Concentration (ppm)		
	< 0.3 ppm	*0.3–0.6 ppm*	*> 0.6 ppm*
6 months–3 years	0.25 mg/day	0	0
3–6 years	0.5 mg/day	0.25 mg/day	0
6–16 years	1.0 mg/day	0.5 mg/day	0

ppm = parts per million.

Table 2–5   Topical Fluoride: Treatment Guidelines[a]

Age/Patient	No/Low Caries	Caries-Prone (2 or more/year)	Rampant Caries (several large lesions)
2 years and under	Fluoride dentrifice (small amount)	Fluoride dentrifice (small amount)	Fluoride dentrifice OTC rinse (1×/day)[b]—use for 1–2 months
2–6 years	Fluoride dentrifice (small amount)	Fluoride dentrifice OTC rinse (1×/day)[b]—use for 1–2 months	Fluoride dentrifice OTC rinse (1×/day)[b] or 0.4% SnF$_2$ gel (1×/day)[b]—use for 1–2 months
6 years and older	Fluoride dentrifice OTC rinse (1×/day) (optional)	Fluoride dentrifice OTC rinse (1×/day) or 0.05% NaF rinse (1×/day) or 0.044% APF rinse (1×/day) or 0.4% SnF$_2$ gel (1–2×/day) or 0.2% NaF rinse (1×/week)	Fluoride dentrifice OTC rinse (1×/day) or 0.05% NaF rinse (1×/day) or 0.044% APF rinse (1×/day) or 0.4% SnF$_2$ gel (1–2×/day) or 0.2% NaF rinse (1×/week) or 1.1% NaF gel (1×/day) or 1.1% APF gel (1×/day)—use until no caries
Patient wearing orthodontic appliances	Fluoride dentrifice OTC rinse (1×/day)	Fluoride dentrifice OTC rinse (1×/day) or 0.5 NaF rinse (1×/day) or 0.2% NaF rinse (1×/week) or 0.4% SnF$_2$ gel (1–2×/day) or 1.1% NaF gel (1×/day)	Fluoride dentrifice OTC rinse (1×/day) or 0.5 NaF rinse (1×/day) or 0.4% SnF$_2$ gel (1–2×/day) or 1.1% NaF gel (1×/day)

NaF = sodium fluoride; OTC = over-the-counter products; SnF$_2$ = stannous fluoride; APF = acidulated phosphate fluoride.
[a]The above are suggested guidelines. The final decision for determining the proper fluoride supplements depends upon the professional's assessment of the patient's needs.
[b]These products are usually not recommended for children under the age of 6 years. Therefore, extreme caution should be taken. Apply these agents in very small amounts with either a cotton-tipped applicator or a small toothbrush.
Based on data from American Dental Association. (1994). *A guide to the use of fluorides for the prevention of dental caries.* Chicago, IL: Author. Wei, S.H.Y. (1985). *Clinical uses of fluorides.* Philadelphia: Lea & Febiger.

when we take vitamins, minerals, or medicine, we need to use the recommended amount of fluoride. The recommended amount is based on our age and how much, if any, fluoride is currently in our drinking water system (see Tables 2–4 and 2–5).

Fluoride Story

The History of Fluoride (A True Story)

Once upon a time, over 80 years ago, a dentist named Frederick McKay moved to Colorado Springs from the East Coast. Because Dr. McKay was trained as a dentist, he wanted to do just what he had done in the east for a living; that is, to help people have healthy mouths and good gums, and to fix cavities or holes in the teeth of those who hadn't learned that brushing away plaque and eating less sugary foods would prevent these cavities from forming. He opened his new office and put out his sign, "Dr. Frederick McKay, D.D.S." (*Write D.D.S. on the board and explain the abbreviation.*)

Dr. McKay hoped people would come to him for help. Soon people did begin to come in for x-rays (which are used to find cavities in between the teeth, and to check formation of permanent teeth in the jaws of younger patients), for checkups, and to have their teeth cleaned. But one thing soon became clear—almost none of them had decay (holes in their teeth). The only people with cavities were those like Dr. McKay who had come from out of town.

Dr. McKay and others asked many questions of these patients. They asked about what they ate and what they drank, trying to find out why they didn't have a problem with cavities like people from other parts of the country did. It took almost 25 years of asking questions and studying the possibilities to discover that the answer was found in the water the people in Colorado were drinking. The water came from the hills in streams from melting snow and it contained a substance called *fluoride. (Write the term on the board.)*

Let me show you a rock like those from the hills in Colorado above where Dr. McKay lived. *(Hold up a rock.)* How do you suppose the fluoride found in this rock gets into the water to make teeth strong? As the water passes over the rocks a tiny, tiny bit of fluoride joins the flowing water from the streams and rivers. Eventually, the water reached the people in Colorado Springs, and they drank this water and the enamel of their teeth got harder and stronger. This was not the very best way to get just the right amount of fluoride, however, because sometimes when the streams were full and running fast there was a different amount of fluoride in the water than in the summer when the water in the streams and rivers was low. After many, many studies and tests, just the right amount of fluoride for water was discovered. One part of fluoride per one million parts of water makes strong teeth that are nice and white.

Many cities have fluoride in their water in this amount, and the people in those cities are very fortunate because just by turning on the faucet and drinking water, cooking foods in this water, and by brushing their teeth with this water they will have stronger, harder teeth with fewer cavities.

(10 minutes)

Guided Practice Activities

This segment may be combined with the preceding instruction/information segment. Visual aids are included at the end of the lesson.

- Utilize small group discussions on various types and uses of fluoride (use the general information presented earlier to stimulate discussion).
- Review types of toothpaste, mouth rinses, and other products that contain fluoride. Display the fluoride ingredients on these product labels. Review the display of fluoride samples used in the anticipatory planning segment of this lesson.
- Identify the types of fluoride through the fluoride family album.
- Present the fluoride family play or story.
- Have the students draw a tooth that received fluoride (see handout).

FLUORIDE FAMILY ALBUM

Create your own album utilizing pictures of fluoride products. This lesson can be used as a lead-in to the fluoride family play, which follows.

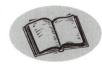

Fluoride Family Story

The Fluoride Family Story

Read the following story to the class (grades K–2) or use as a play (grades 3–6; pick eight students to represent Flo and the members of her family). The narrator can read the story or the family members can read their own dialog.

This is the story of Flo Fluoride and her family.

FAMILY MEMBERS:

Flo (narrator): Fluoride drop
Freddy (father): Fluoride gel
Florence (mother): Fluoride in toothpaste
Fay (sister): Fluoride rinse
Uncle Floyd: Fluoride tablet
Frank and Frannie (cousins to Flo): Fluoride in the water
Grandpa Fester: Fluoride in foods

Flo: My name is Flo Fluoride. You may not know who I am, but I know who you are. My family and I work day and night to keep your teeth healthy and strong. We are invisible while we go about our work, but today I have a special treat for you. You get to meet all of my family. Here I am! I'm hiding inside these fluoride drops that look like water. I'm a fluoride drop. I've helped your teeth since you were just a baby.

Florence: Can you find me? I'm very busy at home. You can usually find me in your toothpaste. I help protect your teeth every time you brush with a fluoride toothpaste. Do you have fluoride in your toothpaste?

Freddy: I work at the dental clinic or office. I'm in the fluoride gel that the dentist or dental hygienist puts on your teeth. Fluoride gel protects your teeth with an invisible shield even after the gel is gone.

Fay: I'm a fluoride rinse. Each time you swish the rinse around in your mouth, fluoride clings to your teeth to protect them. Can you name a fluoride rinse that you can find me in?

Uncle Floyd: I'm a fluoride tablet. Every time you chew a fluoride tablet, I stand guard over your teeth to make them strong.

Cousins Frannie and Frank: We live at the water works but we travel a lot. Sometimes we are added to the water before it goes through town and into your house or the drinking fountain at your school. Every time you drink water with fluoride you are building stronger teeth. Be sure to drink water every day. Is there fluoride in your water?

Grandpa Fester: I'm found in small amounts in the green leafy vegetables, fish, and tuna that you eat to make your bodies big and strong.

Flo: I'm happy that you have been able to meet my family. I'm so proud of all the good work we do for you. The Fluoride family works every day to keep your teeth healthy and strong.

Closure

(2–3 minutes)

- Restate the objectives in question form.
- Check students' knowledge and understanding of the concepts presented.
- If time permits, address any other questions the students may have. Relate the importance of fluoride to dental health.

Leſſon plan / FLUORIDE

GRADE LEVEL _____ ROOM _____

SCHOOL _____ TEACHER _____

TIME REQUIRED (30 MINUTES) _____

Preparation in Classroom _____

_____

_____

_____

_____

_____

Anticipatory Planning _____

_____

_____

_____

_____

_____

_____

_____

Review of Previous Objectives: _____

_____

_____

_____

_____

_____

Three Specific Objectives:

1. _____

_____

2. _____

_____

3. _____

_____

LeSSon plan / **FLUORIDE** *continues*

Information to Be Presented Will Include:

(Topics) _____

_____

_____

_____

_____

_____

(Methods) _____

_____

_____

_____

_____

_____

(Lecture, demonstration, visual aids, group discussion) _____

_____

_____

_____

_____

_____

Guided Practice Activities _____

_____

_____

_____

_____

Closure _____

_____

_____

_____

_____

_____

_____

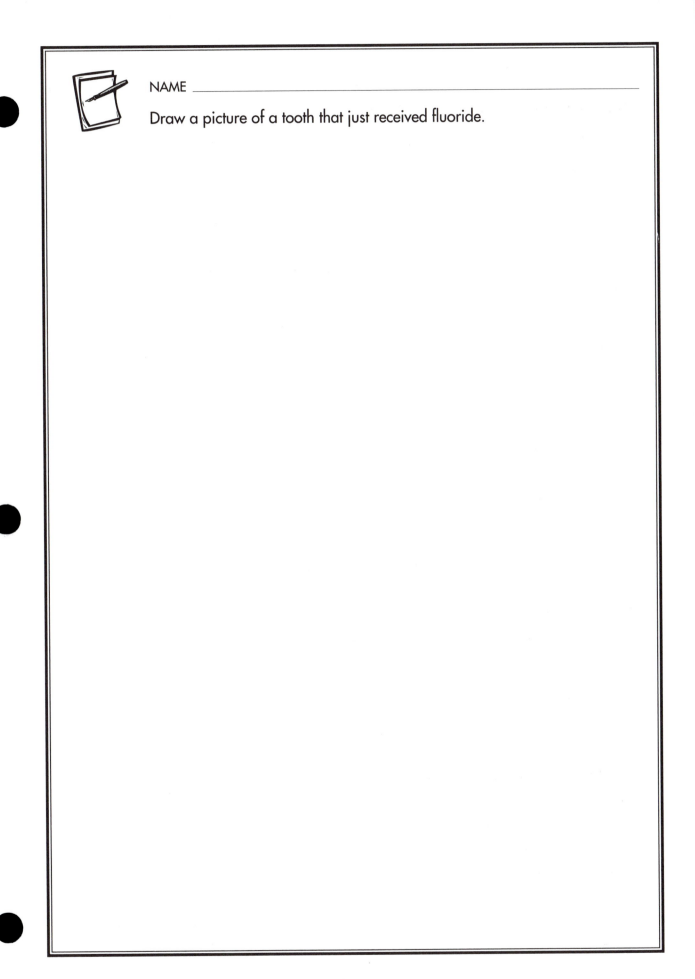

NAME _____

Draw a picture of a tooth that just received fluoride.

the Importance of Plaque Control

Preparation

(5 minutes before beginning lesson)

Assemble the necessary supplies, including disclosing solution or tablets; paper cups; cotton-tipped applicators; small, compact mirrors; and toothbrushes. If appropriate, select students from the class to volunteer for an experiment in which you use a disclosing solution to make the plaque visible.

Anticipatory Planning

(5 minutes)

- Review the previous lesson, if applicable.
- Introduce presenters.
- Describe the goals of today's lesson, the format of information, or general topics to be covered.
- Review classroom rules (K–3), if applicable.

General Objectives by Grade Level

(2–3 minutes)

State specifically no more than three objectives appropriate for the classroom learning level that indicate what the majority of the students will be able to achieve by the completion of the lesson. Keep in mind that for every grade level you advance, the previous grade level objectives could also be used.

Upon completion of this lesson, the student will be able to:

GR	OBJECTIVE
K	Identify that plaque is not pleasant to look at and is not good to have. State that plaque can be disturbed with a soft toothbrush.
1	Describe the dental disease process. Identify where the plaque hides. Identify two consequences of plaque (plaque can hurt your teeth and gums). Define plaque and explain its role in the dental disease process.
2	Identify oral disorders caused by plaque accumulations.
3	List warning signs of gum disease.
4	Include any or all of the above information.
5	Include any or all of the above information.
6	Include any or all of the above information.

Instruction/Information

(10 minutes)

More than one topic may be included or combined with the guided practice segment (10 to 20 minutes). Use as many visuals as possible for grades K–3; group discussion may be more appropriate for grades 4–6. Visual aids are included at the end of the lesson.

- Explain the dental disease process.
- Discuss the consequence of leaving plaque on the teeth and gums.
- Relate the story of the three friends.

Dental disease process

Show the visual of the dental disease process (Fig. 2–1). Discuss how:

Plaque + Sugar = Acid
Acid + Healthy Tooth = Decay (cavities)

Ask why it is important to brush and floss every day. (*Answer:* To remove the plaque the builds up on tooth surfaces.) If the plaque is not removed daily, what can happen? (*Discuss.*) What are the consequences of leaving plaque on the teeth? (*Discuss.*)

Discussion/Visual: Related Topics

Discuss the following topics, using additional visuals that you compile or create:

- Bad breath
- Tooth decay (cavities)
- Gum disease (gingivitis); inflammation around the gums

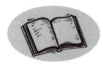

Three Friends Story

The Three Friends

(Developed by the Sacramento County Health Department)

Once upon a time there were three friends. They were sad because they were not like everyone else. Something was missing (see Fig. 2–2). What were they missing? (*Answer:* Teeth, mouth.) Every day they wished they could have teeth and be like everyone else.

One day a good fairy appeared. She said, "I will grant you your wish, but first you must tell me why you want teeth." The first friend said, "I want teeth to help me talk." The second friend said, "I want teeth to help me eat good healthy foods." The third one said, "I want teeth to help me smile."

The good fairy clapped her hands and gave each of them teeth. She told them they were very smart, but they had to promise to brush their teeth every day to keep them healthy. The three friends promised they would brush daily and off they went to school.

As the days passed, they had a good time eating, talking, and smiling . . . but they forgot to brush. Then one day the friends noticed their teeth were getting a yellow film on them and their mouths didn't smell very good. The first friend was starting to have pain in one tooth. The three friends asked the school nurse why the tooth hurt, and she told them about plaque:

- Plaque is a germ that is found on our teeth.
- Plaque can be invisible or yellow.
- Plaque likes to hide on chewing surfaces, between the teeth, along the gums, and on the tongue.
- Plaque germs like to eat sugar. When they eat sugar, they form acid.
- This acid can make holes in our teeth called cavities.
- Plaque also makes our gums red and puffy, and they may bleed.
- We can protect our teeth and keep them healthy by using fluoride, brushing, flossing, eating healthy foods, and going to the dentist.

Now the three friends knew why they needed to take care of their teeth, and they started doing it every day. They went to their new friend, the dentist, who fixed the hole in the first friend's tooth by filling it with silver. Then they saw the dental hygienist, who cleaned their teeth and put fluoride on them.

By brushing their teeth every day, their mouths looked, smelled, and felt clean and fresh.

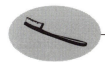

(10 minutes)   ## Guided Practice Activities

This segment may be combined with the preceding instruction/information segment. Visual aids are included at the end of the lesson.

- Have the students draw a picture of plaque attacking a tooth (see handout).
- Disclose the plaque.
- Record the number of teeth that are plaque free.
- Remove the plaque by brushing and/or brushing and flossing.

MAKE THE PLAQUE VISIBLE

Preparation

- State exactly what is going to take place using vocabulary appropriate for the grade level (e.g., first grade—"color the plaque"; fourth grade—"use a special disclosing solution"). Emphasize that this experiment will make the plaque visible. You may have the entire class disclose or only a few volunteers. However, this lesson is more effective when everyone discloses, including the teacher(s).
- Outline the steps you will be using on the black/white board: (1) disclose, (2) find the plaque, (3) brush and floss, (4) final check, and (5) rinse brush.

General Rules

- Don't rinse or drink water until you are told to.
- It's not necessary to look at your friends' plaque to improve your own brushing technique.
- Everyone should remain seated throughout the activity.

Using the Disclosing Solution

1. Dispense the disclosing solution on the students' teeth or hand out tablets that can be chewed by each student, as appropriate to the grade/level (see below).
   a. *Grades K–2:* Place a small amount of disclosing solution in a paper cup. Use a cotton-tipped applicator to paint the disclosing solution on the students' teeth.
   b. *Grades 3–6:* Have the students line up. Place a small amount of disclosing solution on their tongues and have them swish the solution around in their mouths. (Have them return to their seats to evaluate the plaque.)
2. Pass out small, compact mirrors for the students to use to see where the plaque hides, especially in between the teeth. (Be sure to collect the mirrors at the end of the lesson.)
3. Record the number of teeth that are plaque free.

Removing the Plaque

1. Review the dry brushing and flossing (if applicable) technique to be used.
2. Check to see if the plaque is being removed.
3. Rinse the disclosing solution from the toothbrushes.

Pluses for Using Disclosing Solution

- Students and teachers realize plaque is not some obscure thing that dental personnel talk about.

- They see they are not doing a thorough job of brushing and are motivated to brush better and more often as a result.
- They see that dry brushing is effective in removing plaque.
- It gives you an opportunity to identify cases of gross dental neglect.

Closure

(2–3 minutes)
- Restate the objectives in question form.
- Check students' knowledge and understanding of the concepts presented.
- If time permits, address any other questions the students may have.
- Mention that disclosing solution or tablets can be obtained at their local drug store.

Leϳϳon plɑN / PLAQUE CONTROL

GRADE LEVEL _____ ROOM _____

SCHOOL _____ TEACHER _____

TIME REQUIRED (30 MINUTES) _____

Preparation in Classroom _____

_____
_____
_____
_____
_____

Anticipatory Planning _____

_____
_____
_____
_____
_____
_____
_____

Review of Previous Objectives: _____

_____
_____
_____
_____
_____

Three Specific Objectives:

1. _____
_____

2. _____
_____

3. _____
_____

Information to Be Presented Will Include:

(Topics) _____

_____

_____

_____

_____

_____

(Methods) _____

_____

_____

_____

_____

_____

(Lecture, demonstration, visual aids, group discussion) _____

_____

_____

_____

_____

_____

Guided Practice Activities _____

_____

_____

_____

_____

_____

Closure _____

_____

_____

_____

_____

_____

_____

Draw a picture of plaque attacking a healthy tooth.

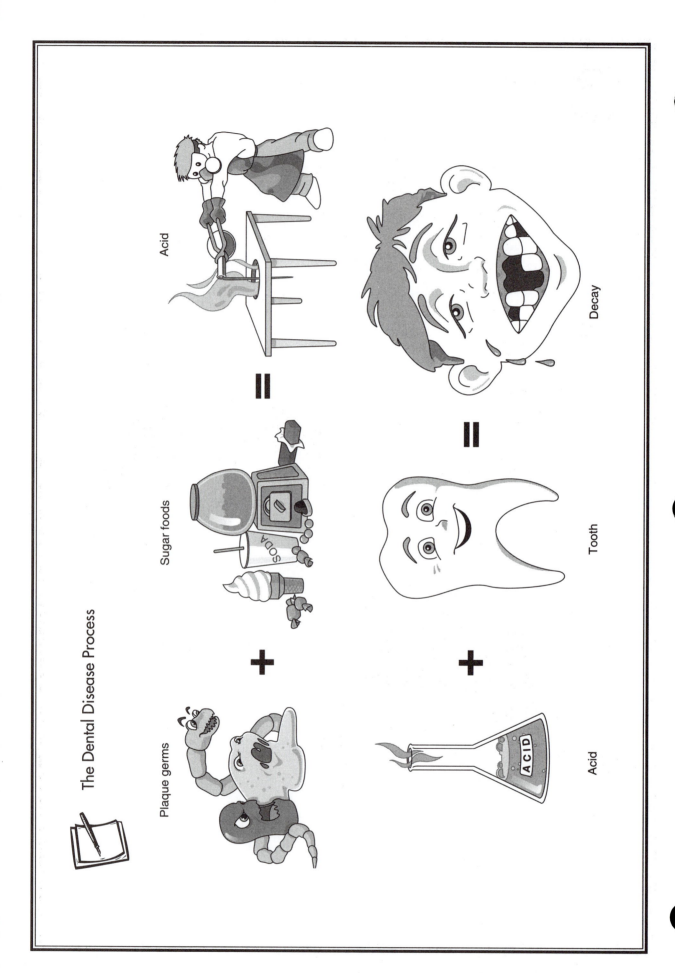

FIGURE 2–1 Dental Disease Process

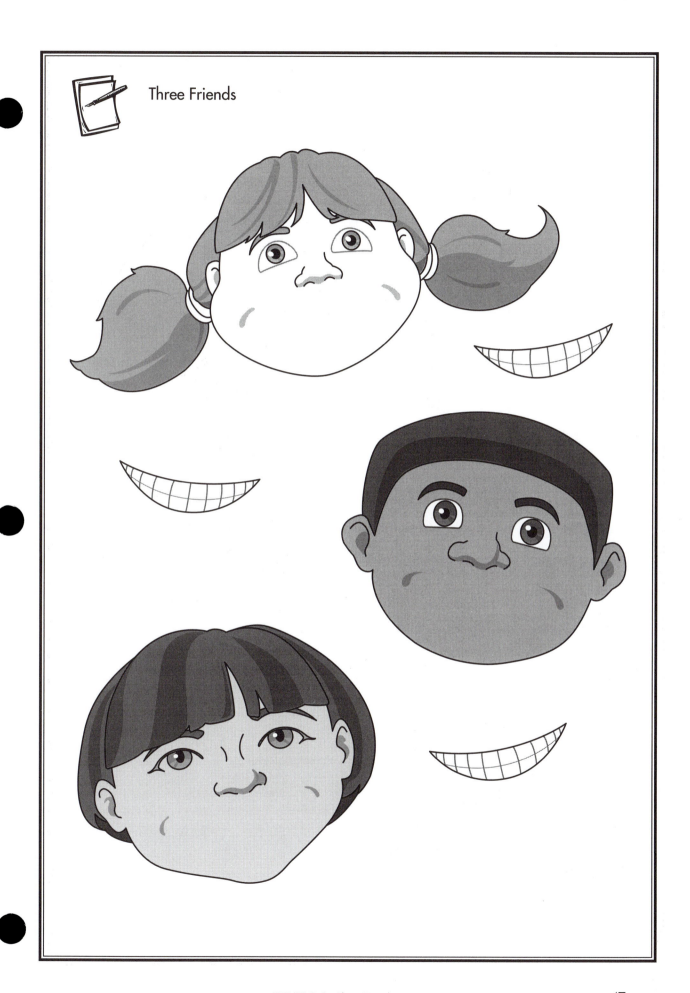

FIGURE 2–2 Three Friends   47

toothbrushing for Good Oral Health

Preparation

(5 minutes before beginning lesson)

Assemble the following items: a large model of teeth; large toothbrush; Styrofoam tooth model (see Section Four); cotton balls to serve as plaque and red felt or marker to indicate inflamed gums; pictures of tooth decay; visual of the decay process; and several storage containers that can be used to store toothbrushes in the classroom.

Anticipatory Planning

(5 minutes)

- Review the previous lesson, if applicable.
- Introduce presenters.
- Describe the goals of today's lesson, the format of information, and general topics to be covered.
- Review classroom rules (K–3), if applicable.

General Objectives by Grade Level

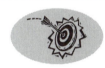

(2–3 minutes)

State specifically no more than three objectives appropriate for the classroom learning level that indicate what the majority of the students will be able to achieve by the completion of the lesson. This lesson may also be incorporated with the objectives and information from the toothbrushing and plaque control lesson. Keep in mind that for every grade level you advance, the previous grade level objectives could also be used.

Upon completion of this lesson, the student will be able to:

GR	OBJECTIVE
K	Describe plaque.
	Describe how plaque can hurt teeth and gums, and areas where plaque hides.
	State the consequences of too much plaque in the mouth.
1	List the characteristics of a good toothbrush and storage recommendations.
2	Demonstrate increased proficiency in brushing teeth.
3	Explain the process of decay, and tell why regular dental visits are important for diagnosing dental problems at their earliest stages.
4	Discuss the signs and causes of periodontal disease, and relate the effects of proper brushing to maintaining the health of the gingiva.
	Discuss the importance to oral health of both personal and professional care.
5	Relate the results of dental neglect to decay and periodontal disease.
	Recognize that each person is responsible for his or her own dental health.
6	Include any or all of the above information.

Instruction/Information

(10 minutes)   More than one topic may be included or combined with the guided practice segment (10 to 20 minutes). Use as many visuals as possible for grades K–3; group discussion may be more appropriate for grades 4–6.

- Discuss plaque (see the previous lesson).
- Explain how brushing daily removes the plaque.

Plaque and your teeth

Discussion/Visual: What Is Plaque?

Plaque is a sticky, clear substance that forms on teeth. It is made of germs and is not good for your teeth. Plaque forms on the teeth every time you eat. If it is not removed, it causes dental diseases. Plaque hides along the gum line (sulcus), in between teeth, and on every surface of the tooth. If plaque is not removed along the gum line, it causes gingivitis (red, puffy gums). If plaque is not removed on the tooth surfaces, it creates acids that eat into the tooth surface, causing cavities (holes in the teeth).

Use visuals to present the following dental disease equations (see the earlier plaque control lesson; Fig. 2–1 for tooth decay and gum disease):

1. Plaque (germs) + Sugar (from the foods we eat) = Acid
   Acid + Healthy tooth = Decay (hole in the tooth)
2. Plaque (germs) + Sugar (from the foods we eat) = Toxin
   Toxin + Healthy gums = Gingivitis (red, puffy gums; gum disease)

Discussion/Visual: Removing the Plaque

Discuss the variety of different types and sizes of toothbrushes that are available. Emphasize the following points:

- Plaque must be removed daily.
- Brush your teeth at least twice a day.
- The most important time to brush is after meals and before going to bed.
- Be sure your toothbrush bristles are soft, straight, and firm. Discard your toothbrush when the bristles become frayed and worn.
- Be sure your toothbrush is the right size for your mouth.
- Never share your toothbrush.

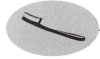

(10 minutes)   ## Guided Practice Activities

This segment may be combined with the preceding instruction/information segment. Visual aids are included at the end of the lesson.

- Illustrate the dry toothbrushing technique in the classroom. Emphasize that toothpaste gives the teeth fluoride protection, but it is not needed to remove the plaque.
- Show different types of toothbrush storage containers and illustrate their use.

CLASSROOM BRUSHING

Preliminary Demonstration/Discussion

1. Demonstrate the proper way to hold a toothbrush.
2. Demonstrate a short, back-and-forth, systematic brushing motion.
3. Describe a sequence for brushing all tooth surfaces (Fig. 2–3).

4. Demonstrate brushing the tongue.
5. Demonstrate proper care of the toothbrush.

Preparation

- Put students' names on brushes.
- Provide toothbrush holders that students can keep at their desks.

General Rules for Brushing

- There should be a toothbrush for each person. Never use anyone else's toothbrush and never allow anyone else to use yours.
- Keep your toothbrush clean. Rinse it under cold running water after brushing. Shake out the excess water and replace it in the holder to air dry.
- Do not store brushes in their original wrappers (box or plastic).
- Replace your toothbrush when it becomes badly worn, or when bristles are frayed or falling out. Never chew on your brush. A brush that is used properly will last much longer than one that is mistreated.
- Never walk around the room with a toothbrush in your mouth. Always carry your brush in your hand to prevent injuries to your mouth that might occur from accidental falls or getting bumped while the toothbrush is in your mouth.

Initial Brushing Session

1. Using the large toothbrush model, demonstrate the proper way to hold a toothbrush.
   a. Grasp the toothbrush with the entire hand, with the thumb pointing toward the bristles.
   b. Use a firm grasp.
2. Pass out the toothbrushes.
3. Have the students demonstrate the proper way to hold the toothbrush.
   a. Have the students hold the toothbrush high in the air.
   b. Quickly check each student.
4. Demonstrate the short, back-and-forth brushing motion outside the mouth.
5. Have each student hold his or her toothbrush in the air and practice moving it in short strokes.
6. Explain the importance of brushing both the teeth and the gums; that is, the toothbrush is placed where the teeth and gums come together. Have students vibrate the bristles of their brushes in place.
7. Have the students demonstrate their proficiency in brushing by dry brushing one quadrant in their mouths. Quickly check each student's technique, watching particularly for proper placement of the toothbrush.
8. When proficiency is achieved, have students brush all quadrants, starting in the outside upper right and moving to the upper left, and then the outside lower left to lower right; then brushing from the inside upper right to upper left; and finally, from the inside lower left to lower right (see Fig. 2–4).
   a. Check for the shortness and direction of the stroke.
   b. Have students brush the biting surfaces and tongue (see Fig. 2–3).
9. Emphasize the importance of systematic brushing so no areas are missed (refer to Fig. 2–4).
10. Instruct students to allow the toothbrush to air dry before putting it away.
11. Tell students to repeat this activity at least twice a day (average brushing time is 2–4 minutes).

TOOTHBRUSH STORAGE CONTAINERS

Show several different types of storage containers for toothbrushes (Fig. 2–5). Emphasize the following points:

- Always let the toothbrush air dry before putting it away.
- Be sure the container is clearly marked with your name.
- Never store a toothbrush in a plastic wrapper.

Closure

(2–3 minutes)

- Restate the objectives in question form.
- Check students' knowledge and understanding of the concepts presented.
- If time permits, address any other questions the students may have.

LeSSon plan / TOOTHBRUSHING

GRADE LEVEL _____ ROOM _____

SCHOOL _____ TEACHER _____

TIME REQUIRED (30 MINUTES) _____

Preparation in Classroom _____
_____
_____
_____
_____
_____

Anticipatory Planning _____
_____
_____
_____
_____
_____
_____
_____

Review of Previous Objectives: _____
_____
_____
_____
_____
_____

Three Specific Objectives:
1. _____
_____
2. _____
_____
3. _____
_____

Information to Be Presented Will Include:

(Topics) _____

_____

_____

_____

_____

_____

(Methods) _____

_____

_____

_____

_____

_____

(Lecture, demonstration, visual aids, group discussion) _____

_____

_____

_____

_____

_____

Guided Practice Activities _____

_____

_____

_____

_____

_____

Closure _____

_____

_____

_____

_____

_____

_____

Brushing

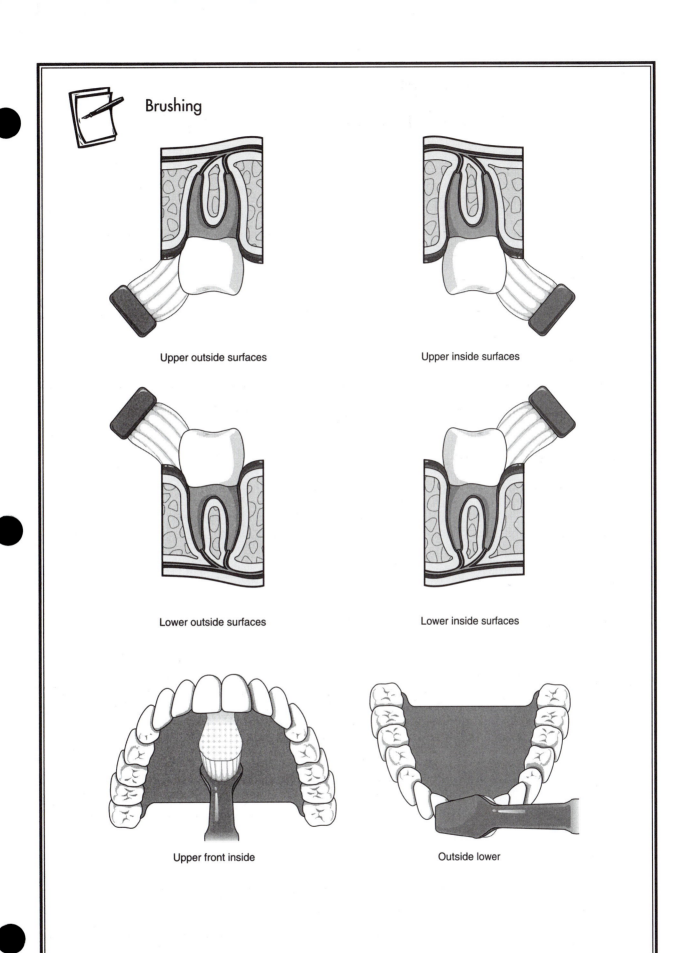

Upper outside surfaces

Upper inside surfaces

Lower outside surfaces

Lower inside surfaces

Upper front inside

Outside lower

FIGURE 2–3 Brushing   55

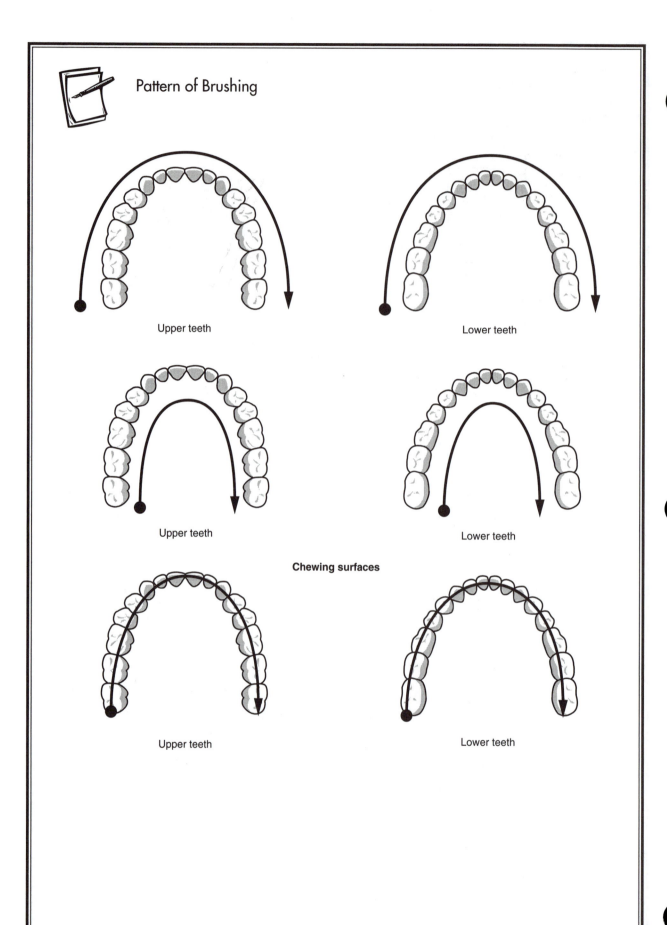

Pattern of Brushing

Upper teeth

Lower teeth

Upper teeth

Lower teeth

Chewing surfaces

Upper teeth

Lower teeth

Toothbrush Storage Ideas

Bulletin board

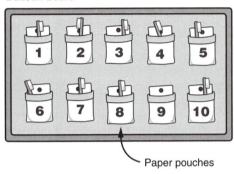

Paper pouches

Mini bins

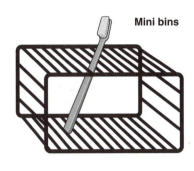

Cup hooks / Nails

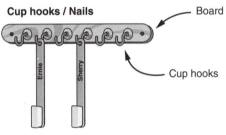

Board

Cup hooks

Commercial toothbrush cover

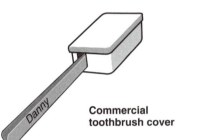

Hanging egg carton

Punch hole on outer edge

Make slit in separator

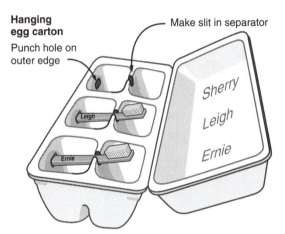

Sherry

Leigh

Ernie

Egg carton can be stored closed, as long as there are holes punched in lid

Egg carton

Punch holes for toothbrushes

Small ventilation holes needed if the toothbrushes face downward

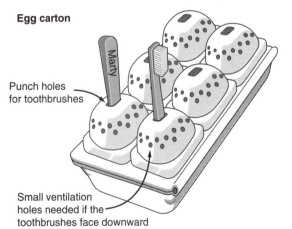

Sponge

Cut slits

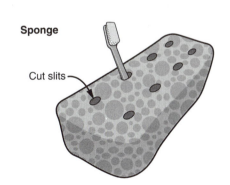

FIGURE 2–5 Toothbrush Storage Ideas 57

$f$lossing for Good Oral Health

Preparation

(5 minutes before beginning lesson) Assemble the following items: several different samples of floss (tape, waxed, unwaxed, flavored, fluoride); large model of teeth; floss holder; and Styrofoam tooth model (see Section Four), with cotton balls to serve as plaque.

Anticipatory Planning

(5 minutes)
- Review the previous lesson, if applicable.
- Introduce presenters.
- Describe the goals of today's lesson, the format of information, or general topics to be covered.
- Review classroom rules (K–3), if applicable.
- Review the dental disease process (see Fig. 2–1).
- Reiterate that toothbrushing does not remove plaque between the teeth.

General Objectives by Grade Level

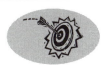

State specifically no more than three objectives appropriate for the classroom learning level that indicate what the majority of the students will be able to achieve by the completion of the lesson. Keep in mind that for every grade level you advance, the previous grade level objectives could also be used.

(2–3 minutes)   Upon completion of this lesson, the student will be able to:

GR	OBJECTIVE
K	Identify dental floss.
1	Describe the function of floss.
2	Explain the importance of floss following an activity that demonstrates its use.
	Relate the lack of interproximal decay and gingival irritation (redness or bleeding) to daily flossing.
3	Demonstrate the ability to floss both front (mesial) and back (distal) sides of the teeth throughout the mouth.
	Identify the gingival sulcus and show how to use dental floss to keep this area clean.
	Demonstrate the use of floss in all areas of the mouth with and without the use of a floss holder.
4	Include any or all of the above information.
5	Include any or all of the above information.
6	Include any or all of the above information.

Instruction/Information

(10 minutes) More than one topic may be included or combined with the guided practice segment (10 to 20 minutes). Use as many visuals as possible for grades K–3; group discussion may be more appropriate for grades 4–6.

- Discuss the importance of daily flossing.
- Describe the different types of floss available.

General information

First, ask students how we might remove plaque from between the teeth. Explain how the brush won't fit there. Next, use real floss or yarn to remove plaque from the large tooth model. Ask students: (1) if they have tried flossing before; and (2) how many have floss in their home or have seen their parents floss.

Explain the different types of floss available: tape, waxed, unwaxed, flavored (colored), and fluoride. Show samples of each. Demonstrate flossing technique by using real floss on your own front teeth.

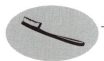

(10 minutes)

Guided Practice Activities

This segment may be combined with the preceding instruction/information segment. Visual aids are included at the end of the lesson.

- Relate the story of the Big King.
- Perform the yarn activity for grades K–2.
- Demonstrate flossing in the classroom for grades 3–6.

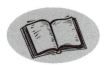

Flossing Story

The Big King

To be told after flossing is taught and before practice to reinforce flossing concepts.

Make two tooth costumes. Using a white pillow case, draw a large happy molar on one side and a sad molar on the other (see Fig. 2–6). Provide prince and princess crowns and a toothbrush.

Once upon a time in a faraway land, there lived a great BIG king who had great BIG teeth. The king lived in a great BIG palace and had many servants. One day the king was looking at his teeth and saw lots of plaque. There was plaque on the sides of his teeth and even in between. The king was really sad; the teeth were sad, too! *(Why?)*

The king wanted his teeth clean, but he didn't know how to clean them. He called out, "Servants! Servants! Come clean my teeth." The servants could not believe the king would ask such a thing. They all agreed to say no to the king. They said, "No way! We clean the floors; we clean the windows; we make the food. We will not clean your teeth, too!" This made the king angry, and he told the servants, "You are all fired! Go home!" Now the king was all alone and he still did not know how to clean his teeth. He sat and thought and thought until he fell fast asleep (zzzzz!).

In the middle of the night, along came a fairy princess. *(Pick a girl from the class to be the princess; give her a crown and a toothbrush.)* The princess thought that maybe if she brushed the plaque away, the king might call the servants back to the palace and the king and his teeth would be happy. But there was one place her brush would not fit. Does anyone know where that was? *(In between.)*

The princess wasn't easily discouraged. She called on her friend, who was a prince. *(Pick a boy from the class to be the prince; give him a crown and yarn for floss.)* He had a very special piece of string. What's the name of this special string? *(Dental floss.)* The prince moved the floss up and down, resting it on the side of the king's teeth, to remove the plaque. He flossed all of the king's teeth—front teeth, molars, on top, and on the bottom.

The prince and princess were all done, and just in time—the king was about to wake up. The king opened his eyes and called out, "Where's my breakfast?" Then he remembered that he was all alone. Just at that moment, he looked at his teeth and saw that they were sparkling clean. That made the king so happy, do you know what he did? He called all the servants back to the palace that day and said, "Today you will all have fun. Nobody works today."

The king thought that the servants cleaned his teeth. Let's not tell him, okay? Because the servants, the prince, and princess, the king, and his teeth all lived happily ever after.

Follow-up Activity: The Big King

Have students in grades 3–6 practice flossing. Supplement with the yarn activity for grades K–2.

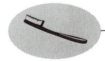

Guided Practice Activities

FLOSSING YARN ACTIVITY (FOR GRADES K–2)

Directions

1. Cut pieces of yarn that are approximately 12 inches long and pass them out to all students.
2. Explain the purpose of flossing, demonstrate flossing, and show students real dental floss.
3. Introduce the activity by telling students that the yarn will represent floss and their fingers, teeth.
4. Model the activity first by having one adult demonstrate flossing on a hand (representing five teeth) that is held up by another adult.

Winding the "Floss"

1. Instruct students to hold the "floss" like a bicycle handle. They should leave a little "floss" sticking out of each fist.
2. Have them point two index fingers straight out, then to the floor, then toward themselves, then to the ceiling. Have them pinch the "floss" with their index finger and thumb.
3. Tell students to "floss" carefully on both sides of their partner's "teeth" (fingers). They should floss one hand first, then the other.

Do not begin the activity until each partner has a piece of floss. Talk the students through the winding and flossing, and when the students are finished flossing both of their partners' hands, have them hold their floss up high. When all are ready (all hands are raised with floss), instruct the students to exchange roles.

FINGER FLOSSING (FOR GRADES 3–6)

Preliminary Demonstration/Discussion

1. Demonstrate flossing on a large tooth model. Explain the use of the finger flossing chart (see Fig. 2–7).
2. Measure and tear off floss from individual containers and pass out to students. Pieces should be about 18 inches long.

3. Explain that when flossing we must be careful not to injure the gums. If we do, they might bleed. (Use the analogy of getting a paper cut.)

General Rules for Flossing

- Don't jam the floss between your teeth.
- Always be in control of the floss.
- To floss your lower teeth, put one finger on the inside of your teeth.
- To floss your upper teeth, put the pointer finger inside to guide the floss.
- Establish a path or journey so that no teeth are missed.
- Be sure to hug the side of the next tooth and slide the floss up and down the side of that tooth.
- Throw the floss away when you are through.

(2–3 minutes)

Closure

- Restate the objectives in question form.
- Check students' knowledge and understanding of the concepts presented.
- If time permits, address any other questions the students may have.

Lesson plan / FLOSSING

GRADE LEVEL _____ ROOM _____

SCHOOL _____ TEACHER _____

TIME REQUIRED (30 MINUTES) _____

Preparation in Classroom _____

_____

_____

_____

_____

_____

Anticipatory Planning _____

_____

_____

_____

_____

_____

_____

_____

Review of Previous Objectives: _____

_____

_____

_____

_____

_____

Three Specific Objectives:

1. _____

_____

2. _____

_____

3. _____

_____

Information to Be Presented Will Include:

(Topics) _____

_____

_____

_____

_____

_____

(Methods) _____

_____

_____

_____

_____

_____

(Lecture, demonstration, visual aids, group discussion) _____

_____

_____

_____

_____

_____

Guided Practice Activities _____

_____

_____

_____

_____

Closure _____

_____

_____

_____

_____

_____

_____

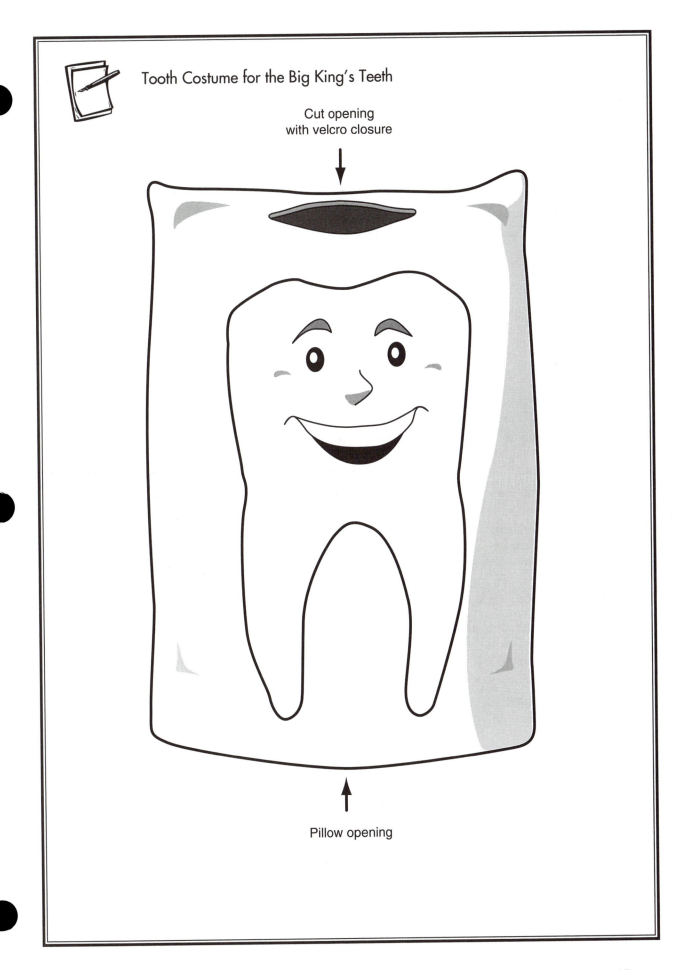

FIGURE 2–6 Tooth costume for the Big King's teeth.

Finger Flossing

Dental floss helps get your teeth really clean by removing plaque from between your teeth and under the gums.

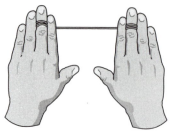

1. Wrap about 18 inches of floss around your middle fingers.

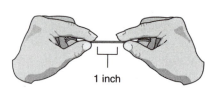

1 inch

2. "Pinch an inch" of floss.

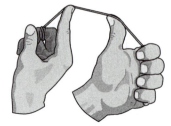

3. Use your thumb and index finger to guide the floss between your upper teeth.

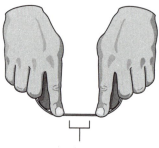

1 inch

4. Use your index fingers to guide the floss between your lower teeth.

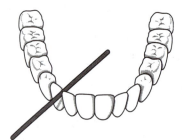

5. Work the floss gently between your teeth.

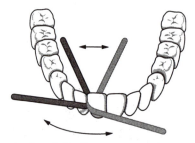

6. Bend the floss around the tooth in a C or U shape.

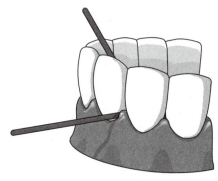

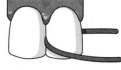

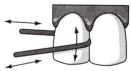

7. Now pull the floss against the tooth. Move the floss gently under the gum until you feel resistance.

8. Holding the floss firmly against your tooth, scrape the plaque from the side of your tooth, moving the floss up and down five times. Be sure to floss both sides of each tooth.

Move to a clean area of floss after every two or three teeth.

FIGURE 2–7   Finger Flossing

Nutrition and Healthy Teeth

Preparation

(5 minutes before beginning lesson)

Assemble pictures or cards of foods; a picnic or a class party menu; a variety of packaged foods and snacks, some of which contain sugar, others of which are sugar-free; a chart of the food pyramid; and a 1-lb box of sugar. Bring information about nutrition from your local dairy council.

Anticipatory Planning

(5 minutes)

- Review the previous lesson, if applicable.
- Introduce presenters.
- Describe the goals of today's lesson, the format of information, and general topics to be covered.
- Review classroom rules (K–3), if applicable.
- Survey the class about current food choices. (Ask: "What did you eat for breakfast?")
- Review the dental disease process (see Fig. 2–1).

General Objectives by Grade Level

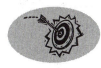

(2–3 minutes)

State specifically no more than three objectives appropriate for the classroom learning level that indicate what the majority of the students will be able to achieve by the completion of the lesson. Keep in mind that for every grade level you advance, the previous grade level objectives could also be used.

Upon completion of this lesson, the student will be able to:

GR	OBJECTIVE
K/1	State that a variety of foods are needed for health and to build strong bodies. Choose a variety of foods that are good for teeth. Identify the food groups and their place in the food pyramid.
2	State why foods at the top of the pyramid should be used sparingly.
3	Include any or all of the above information.
4	Include any or all of the above information.
5	Include any or all of the above information.
6	Include any or all of the above information.

Instruction/Information

(10 minutes)

More than one topic may be included or combined with the guided practice segment (10 to 20 minutes). Use as many visuals as possible for grades K–3; group discussion may be more appropriate for grades 4–6.

- Explain why good nutrition is important.
- Present the food pyramid.
- Review the recommended daily requirements.
- Discuss the importance of dental nutrition.
- Relate the facts and myths of dental nutrition.

General information

The food pyramid illustrates the principles of a healthy diet recommended by professionals and national health organizations. A balanced diet is important in preventing cavities; however, cavities are also the results of what we eat and how often these foods are eaten.

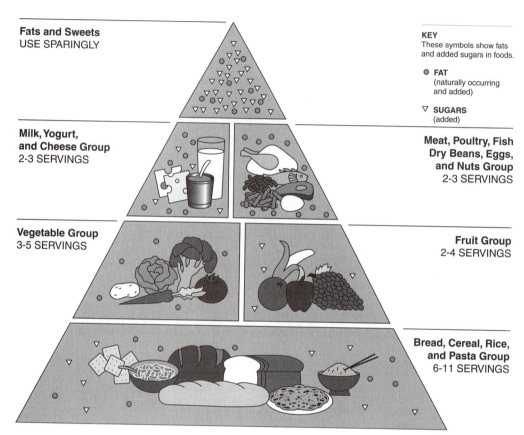

Fats and Sweets
USE SPARINGLY

Milk, Yogurt, and Cheese Group
2-3 SERVINGS

Meat, Poultry, Fish Dry Beans, Eggs, and Nuts Group
2-3 SERVINGS

Vegetable Group
3-5 SERVINGS

Fruit Group
2-4 SERVINGS

Bread, Cereal, Rice, and Pasta Group
6-11 SERVINGS

KEY
These symbols show fats and added sugars in foods.

● **FAT** (naturally occurring and added)

▽ **SUGARS** (added)

When we eat, particles of foods can become trapped on or between tooth surfaces. When complex carbohydrate foods such as bread, corn flakes, pasta, crackers, and potato chips are allowed to remain in the mouth without brushing, the bacteria that live in the mouth break down these starches into sugars. These sugars, in turn, are converted into acids that can eat away at tooth enamel. Frequent snacking leaves food on our teeth longer; thus, it is more apt to begin the decay process (see Fig. 2–1). For this reason, sugars and starches are best reserved for mealtime when increased saliva production helps to neutralize the acid attack.

Acid-producing foods include:

- Cakes
- Candy
- Cookies
- Cough drops
- Doughnuts
- Gelatin dessert
- Gum
- Honey
- Jams
- Jellies
- Liqueurs
- Mints

- Molasses
- Pies
- Popsicles
- Soft drinks
- Syrup
- Table sugar

The texture of some foods causes them to be retained in the mouth longer than others. For instance, hard candies and chocolates dissolve and clear the mouth quickly. However, raisins and sticky foods such as caramels, gumdrops, or peanut butter remain on the teeth for longer periods of time unless brushed off.

Research has shown that certain foods have anti-cavity power; that is, they reduce the amount of acid exposure to the teeth. These foods are more dentally sound because they fight plaque and neutralize the acid-producing bacteria. Examples include:

- Hard cheese (e.g., Jack, Cheddar, Swiss)
- Raw fruits and vegetables
- Peanuts and cashews

It is important to alternate these dentally preferred snacks in our daily diet. This provides a variety of choices and ensures a balanced intake of nutritious foods.

The food pyramid

Each of the food groups in the food pyramid provides some, but not all, of the nutrients we need each day. Foods in one group can't replace those in another group; therefore, no one food group is more important than any another. However, the small tip of the pyramid shows "extras," such as oils and sweets, that offer few, if any, nutrients relative to the calories, fat, or sugar they contain.

The number of servings from the different groups varies. These recommended daily servings ensure that we consume adequate nutrients while moderating the amount of fat, sugar, and calories in our diets (Table 2–6).

This information can be modified for children in grades K–3 and 4–6 as noted below.

Grades K–3

The pyramid helps us to learn about the foods we need to have energy and healthy bodies. More of our servings should come from foods at the bottom of the pyramid. But it is still important to eat foods from all the food groups. As long as

Table 2–6 Recommended Daily Requirements

Food Group	Number of Servings	
	Age 5–9 years	Age 9 years–Adult
Bread	6–9	6–11
Vegetables	3–4	3–5
Fruit	2–3	2–4
Milk	2–3	2–3
Meat	2–3	2–3
Extras (fats, oils, and sugars)[a]		Use sparingly

[a]Added to enrich foods by adding variety and taste.
Note: The food pyramid is built from the bottom up; thus, the bread and cereals builds a foundation for our bodies to grow. We need these foods for energy.

we're getting enough foods from the food groups to fill our pyramids it's okay to eat some "extras" in moderation or with our meals.

Grades 4–6

The pyramid helps us choose a variety of foods in the proper amounts to keep our bodies healthy. Each food group gives us different essential nutrients, so it's important to eat foods from all the food groups every day. When foods are eaten in the recommended amounts, we can be sure we'll get our daily requirements for the nutrients we need to grow and feel great. More of our total servings should come from the bottom group, but that doesn't take the place of servings from the other groups. Eating "extras" is okay as long as they aren't eaten instead of foods we need to fill up our pyramids. That's because these "extras" contain few if any nutrients. By following the recommended servings from each group, we also keep from getting too much fat and sugar.

Follow-up Activities: The Food Pyramid

- Have students plan a menu using food cards. See how many foods from the pyramid fit into three meals.
- Have students identify foods that would be good snacks.
- Have students tell what they brought for lunch. Have the class identify which foods fit into which groups in the pyramid.
- Review the foods and serving sizes required for each group by building the "Great Food Pyramid."
- Ask students to keep track of the foods they eat for 1 week. At the next lesson, ask whether they met the daily requirements of the food pyramid.
- Present the information on tips for healthy class parties found in Table 2–7.

Dental nutrition

Although sugar is an essential part of the diet, refined sugar consumption among Americans has skyrocketed out of control. Because sugar has a primary role in dental diseases, it should be apparent that nutrition education is a vital part of dental education.

Healthy teeth are possible for most people if knowledge of dental disease is used to alter unhealthy habits. Refined sugar is difficult to eliminate totally from the diet, but the form, frequency, and timing of sugar consumption can be altered. By improving nutritional knowledge and fostering a change in habits, we can help assure better dental health for most people.

Discussion: Facts and Myths of Dental Nutrition

Present the following facts:

- The average American will consume approximately his or her own weight in sugar in 1 year.
- The longer sugar stays in the mouth and the more frequently sweets are eaten, the more opportunity acids have to form.
- Sweets are less harmful to the teeth if eaten with a main meal rather than between meals.
- Liquid sweets are somewhat less harmful than sticky sweets.
- Table sugar is more harmful than sugars that occur naturally in fruits and milk.

Table 2–7 Tips for Class Parties

Goals

1. Eliminate or reduce nonnutritious foods and those that are not dentally safe.
2. Eat foods that aren't dentally safe with meals.
3. Eat foods that are nutritious and dentally safe for between-meal snacks.
4. Brush after eating.

Serve Nutritious Snacks and Beverages

Snacks
    Fresh fruits
    Vegetables with dips
    Cheese cubes
    Wheat crackers
    Popcorn
    Whole-grain breads, corn bread
    Cookies (sweetened with fructose; made with oatmeal, carob chips, and/or whole wheat
       flour)
Beverages
    Sparkling cider
    Unsweetened fruit juices
    Sparkling water
    Eggnog
    Protein drinks

Be Aware of Outside Influences Affecting Nutritional Choices

Peer pressure

Mass media

School

Parents

Grocery stores

Debunk the following myths:

- Eating apples, celery, and carrots *does not* aid significantly in plaque removal.
- Brushing your teeth or rinsing your mouth immediately after eating sweets is not an effective means of inhibiting acid formation.
- Natural sugars such as honey, molasses, corn sweetener, and raw sugar have the same acid-producing effects as does refined sugar.

(Note: *All* of the above statements are false.)

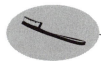

(10 minutes) ## Guided Practice Activities

This segment may be combined with the instruction/information segment. Visual aids are included at the end of the lesson.

- Perform the hidden sugar demonstration.
- Demonstrate how students can read the labels of various food products to identify those containing sugar.
- Have students find the supersnack words in the puzzle (see handout).

- Relate the story of Happy Tooth and Sad Tooth.
- Have the students draw Happy Tooth and Sad Tooth (see handout).

HIDDEN SUGAR DEMONSTRATION

First, relate the average sugar intake per adult per year in the United States (about 135 lbs). Show a 1-lb or 5-lb box of sugar to illustrate. Next, state the amount of refined sugar our bodies require (zero). Emphasize that we get all the sugar we need from the sugar found naturally in fruits and vegetables. Explain the role of sugar in tooth decay (see Fig. 2–1).

The following activity helps to illustrate how we manage to consume so much sugar, often without realizing it, during our daily meals and snacks. Describe a hypothetical breakfast, lunch, and afternoon snack of a school student (see Table 2–8). Write the menu items on the black/white board. Place a teaspoonful of table sugar into a clear glass, spoonful by spoonful, to indicate the amount of sugar in each item of the sample menu. Have students calculate the amount of sugar in each food item. (Note: 1 tsp = 3 grams.)

READING THE LABELS

The following activities can help increase students' awareness of the sugar found in the food they eat each day:

1. Assemble a variety of packaged foods and snacks, some of which contain sugar, others of which are sugar free. Explain that all packaged foods are required by law to list ingredients, which are always displayed in order of their amount by weight in the product. Ask students to explain what a "junk food" is. (*Answer:* A junk food is defined as a food that contains more sugar than nutrients.) Tell students that junk foods can be identified by looking at food product labels. Junk foods are those foods that list sugar or a word meaning sugar as the first or second ingredient.
2. Show a poster of or list on the blackboard various words that indicate sugar: syrup, honey, molasses, sweeteners, any word ending in "-ose." Follow up this activity with label reading.
3. Ask students how we can determine whether a food has sugar in it. (*Answer:* Read labels, read recipes, and taste for sweetness.)

Table 2–8   Hidden Dietary Sugar

Meal	Item (1 serving)	Sugar (tsp)
Breakfast	Fruit Loops cereal	4
	Doughnut	6
	Hot cocoa	6
	Tang	8
Lunch	Skippy peanut butter	1
	Jelly	3
	White bread (2 slices)	2.5
	Potato chips	1
	Pepsi	10
	Cookies (2)	6
Snack	Chocolate cake	10
	High-C drink	7

4. Have students find the supersnack words (words without sugar) in the word puzzle (see handout). Encourage students to choose a sugar-free snack after school, at least for the day. Ask students to promise to read the ingredients on the next packaged product they eat.

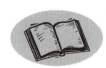

Happy Tooth and Sad Tooth Story

Happy Tooth and Sad Tooth

Assemble the following supplies:

2 pieces of 18- by 24-inch easel paper, to be taped to the blackboard or pinned to the wall
Markers in two colors
Pictures of food cut out of magazines and newspaper ads

Today's story is about two molar teeth. Do any of you know which teeth are molars? They are the teeth way in the back of your mouth. Put your tongue on your very back tooth. Feel what a big tooth it is? Some of you have brand new molars there. These are permanent teeth that won't fall out. They are supposed to last forever, so we must take good care of them.

The first story is about a happy, healthy molar. This tooth uses fluoride to be strong, it brushes to get rid of plaque, it flosses to keep the sides clean and healthy, and it visits the dentist regularly. This tooth eats good foods like fruits, vegetables, and cheese. *(Have the class suggest some other good foods.)* It looks good and feels good because it takes good care of itself. This tooth will be easy to draw because we all know it. Do you know its name? *(Happy Tooth.)*

Now I'm going to tell you about another molar. This tooth forgets to brush, floss, or use fluoride. It doesn't feel well and it doesn't look well. What is its name? *(Sad Tooth.)* Can you imagine what kinds of food Sad Tooth eats. *(Have students name a few.)*

Follow-up Activities: Happy Tooth and Sad Tooth

1. Have the students draw Happy Tooth and Sad Tooth, using the following script:
   a. Draw Happy Tooth first. Start with the crown. *(Describe what the crown is.)* Next draw the roots, which are the feet and legs of a tooth. *(Explain that the roots hold the teeth in our mouths; that permanent teeth have long roots; and that molars have two or three roots.)* Put the eyes on Happy Tooth *(have the students choose happy or sad expression)*, nose, mouth *(happy or sad)*, arms *(strong or weak)*, and cape *(smooth or torn)*. Happy Tooth takes good care of himself and eats nutritious foods.
   b. Now lets draw Sad Tooth. Is it healthy? Is it happy? How will we begin? What does Sad Tooth's crown look like? *(Draw a molar with holes in the top. Have the students complete the drawing as for Happy Tooth, adding arms, roots, face, cape, etc.)*
2. Place the pictures of food you've cut out of magazines and newspaper ads in a lunch bag. Half of the pictures should be of good foods, the other half of bad foods. Ask the class to indicate which are good food choices and which are bad food choices. Tape the pictures around the appropriate tooth picture. Leave the pictures in the classroom to help remind students to make good food choices. Tell them to bring in pictures to add around the appropriate tooth. Emphasize how Sad Tooth could become happy.

Closure

(2–3 minutes)

- Restate the objectives in question form.
- Check students' knowledge and understanding of the concepts presented.
- If time permits, address any other questions the students may have.

Lesson plan / NUTRITION

GRADE LEVEL _____ ROOM _____

SCHOOL _____ TEACHER _____

TIME REQUIRED (30 MINUTES) _____

Preparation in Classroom _____
_____
_____
_____
_____
_____

Anticipatory Planning _____
_____
_____
_____
_____
_____
_____
_____
_____

Review of Previous Objectives: _____
_____
_____
_____
_____
_____

Three Specific Objectives:

1. _____
_____

2. _____
_____

3. _____
_____

Information to Be Presented Will Include:

(Topics) _____

_____

_____

_____

_____

_____

(Methods) _____

_____

_____

_____

_____

_____

(Lecture, demonstration, visual aids, group discussion) _____

_____

_____

_____

_____

_____

Guided Practice Activities _____

_____

_____

_____

_____

_____

Closure _____

_____

_____

_____

_____

_____

_____

_____

NAME _____

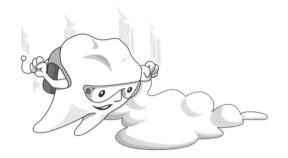

Find the supersnack words (words without sugar) in this puzzle. (Hint: Words may be found across, backward, down, or diagonally.)

M	C	E	L	E	R	Y	P	Z	S
B	I	T	H	E	E	T	E	G	G
U	P	L	Y	S	O	Z	A	M	T
Z	V	R	K	G	O	N	N	R	P
A	P	P	L	E	R	P	U	H	E
A	T	A	I	O	U	J	T	C	G
R	A	F	C	H	E	E	S	E	N
D	C	P	V	K	D	H	B	P	A
S	O	C	A	R	R	O	T	Q	R
P	W	J	A	Z	Z	I	P	M	O

Can you find the following words?

Apple	Carrot	Cheese	Taco
Celery	Popcorn	Egg	Peanuts
Milk	Orange	Pizza	

77

Draw pictures of Happy Tooth and the foods it would eat.

dental Safety and Oral Injury Prevention

Preparation

(5 minutes before beginning lesson)

Display a dental emergency kit (easy to make), dental emergency procedures wall chart, protective equipment (mouth guard, face protector, etc.), and safety signs.

Anticipatory Planning

(5 minutes)

- Review the previous lesson, if applicable.
- Introduce presenters.
- Describe the goals of today's lesson, the format of information, and general topics to be covered.
- Review classroom rules (K–3), if applicable.
- Survey the class about how many students wear protective gear when playing sports. (Ask: "Why is safety important to our teeth?")

General Objectives by Grade Level

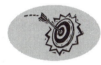

(2–3 minutes)

State specifically no more than three objectives appropriate for the classroom learning level that indicate what the majority of the students will be able to achieve by the completion of the lesson. Keep in mind that for every grade level you advance, the previous grade level objectives could also be used.

Upon completion of this lesson, the student will be able to:

GR	OBJECTIVE
K	Name the dental safety rules.
1	Explain what do if a tooth is accidentally knocked out.
2	Explain the contents and purpose of a dental emergency kit.
3	Describe what to do for various dental emergencies.
4	Include any or all of the above information.
5	Include any or all of the above information.
6	Include any or all of the above information.

Instruction/Information

(15–20 minutes)

More than one topic may be included or combined with the guided practice segment (10 to 20 minutes). Use as many visuals as possible for grades K–3; group discussion may be more appropriate for grades 4–6.

- Present the dental safety rules.
- Describe the contents of a dental emergency kit.
- Discuss first aid for dental emergencies.
- Explain the different types of protective equipment that should be worn for various sports and play activities.

Dental safety rules

Use discussion, visual aids such as posters, or a guided practice activity to teach the following safety rules. Emphasize that many injuries that involve the teeth are preventable (see Fig. 2–8). By following good safety rules, you can prevent these types of injuries to your teeth.

Twelve Rules for Dental Safety

1. *Water/Puddles:* Always walk, don't run, around pools; be careful when walking on rainy days.
2. *Fighting:* This is not the way to solve problems. It's better to walk away, ask for help, or talk it out with the person.
3. *Stairs:* Walk, don't run, up and down stairs. Hold onto the banister. Don't slide down the banister.
4. *Seat belts:* Keep belts fastened at all times when riding in a car.
5. *Chewing on things:* Hard objects such as ice can fracture tooth. Sucking on lemons can also damage the teeth.
6. *Baseball games:* Don't swing or throw the bat when someone is standing near you. Always wear a helmet. Put the glove in front of your face when catching the ball.
7. *Swing sets:* Don't stand or jump on or off the swing. Be careful of others standing close to your swing.
8. *Reaching for things in high places:* Don't stand on a chair with wheels. Ask an adult for help.
9. *Ladder:* Check the equipment before climbing on it. Be sure a parent is nearby.
10. *Rocks:* Watch where you're walking. It's easy to trip over rocks or other objects when you're not looking in front of you.
11. *Drinking fountain:* Don't push or shove or fool around in line while at the drinking fountain.
12. *Objects that don't belong in your mouth:* Objects such as pencils, paper clips, and coins can break or chip your teeth. The only things you should put in your mouth are food, toothbrushes, and floss.

Dental emergency kit

Every home and classroom should have a dental emergency kit available so that proper dental first aid can be administered when injuries occur. Many schools already have some of these items as part of their general first-aid kit. Be sure to provide the name(s) of a local dentist who can be contacted in case of an emergency if a family does not have one.

The kit should contain the following supplies*:

- Cotton and cotton swabs: To clean the injury
- Dental floss, interdental cleaner, and toothpicks: To remove objects from between the teeth
- Dental wax or candle: To stop irritation to cheeks or gums from a chipped tooth or orthodontic wires
- Handkerchief, tie, or towel: To immobilize a broken jaw
- Ice pack: To help reduce swelling
- Medications (consult the school nurse or health aide)
- Hank's solution, Save-a-Tooth, cold milk, or sterile gauze or a clean cloth: To provide temporary storage for a knocked-out tooth

*Adapted with permission from *Prevention of Oral Injuries* Flip Chart, sponsored by the Dental Health Foundation and California Department of Health Services, Dental Health Section, Sacramento, CA; courtesy of Andrea Azevedo.

Dental emergency procedures

Teachers and students should know how to provide first aid for the most common dental emergencies. Present information on simple first-aid techniques for the following dental problems and emergencies.

Bitten Tongue

Apply direct pressure to the site of the irritation, and cover the bleeding area with a sterile or clean cloth. If swelling is present, apply cold compresses. If the bleeding doesn't stop readily or the bite is severe, take the child to the hospital emergency department.

Broken Tooth

Try to clean dirt or debris from the injured area with warm water. Place a cold compress on the face next to the injured tooth to minimize swelling. Take the child to the dentist immediately.

Knocked-out Tooth

Place the tooth in water, Hank's solution, or a Save-a-Tooth container, or wrap it in a clean, wet cloth. *Do not clean the tooth!* Take the child and the tooth to the dentist immediately.

Objects Wedged Between the Teeth

Try to remove the object with dental floss. Guide the floss in carefully so as not to cut the gums. If unsuccessful, take the child to a dentist. *Do not* try to remove wedged objects using a sharp or pointed object.

Orthodontia Problems

Take the child to the orthodontist if:

- A wire is causing irritation
- A wire is embedded in the cheek, tongue, or gum tissue

Do not attempt to remove loose or broken appliances.

Possible Fractured Jaw

If a fracture is suspected, immobilize the jaw by any means (handkerchief, towel) and take the child to the hospital emergency department immediately.

Toothache

Rinse the mouth vigorously with warm water to clean out debris. Use dental floss to remove any food that might be trapped within the cavity. If swelling is present, apply cold compresses to the outside of the cheek. *(Do not use heat.)* Do not place aspirin on the gum tissue or aching tooth. Take the child to the dentist.

Protective equipment

Emphasize that protective equipment should be worn for all sports and play activities that can result in dental or other injuries. Students should also be aware of simple safety measures that can prevent injuries during these activities. Present the information in Table 2–9. Have the students come up with other protective equipment items that should be worn during sports or play activities. As a related activity, you could have students dress up in some of the protective equipment.

Table 2–9   Protective Equipment and Safety Tips for Sports/Play Activities

Sport/Play Activity	Prevention
Football	Wear mouth guard, helmet
Baseball	Wear catcher's mask, helmet
Basketball	Wear mouth guard
Running games	Never trip; watch out for dangerous objects
Swimming and diving	Don't push; don't run; use a ladder
Tree climbing	Watch footing
Bicycling	Wear helmet; use care on wet roads and dirt
Skateboarding	Wear mouth guard, helmet, wrist and knee bands
Roller skating	Control speed; wear helmet, wrist and knee bands
Playground	Don't push or trip
Hill climbing	Check for firm footing
Soccer	Wear mouth guard, shin guards

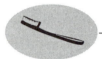

(10 minutes)   ## Guided Practice Activities

This segment may be combined with the preceding instruction/information segment. Visuals aids are included at the end of the lesson.

- Make a dental emergency kit for the classroom. Have students list the items to be included in the kit (see handout).
- Have students review the Play Safe worksheet (Fig. 2–8). Students in grades K–3 can color in the pictures of each safety problem. Ask the students to explain what the teeth are doing wrong in each picture.
- Have students list the safety rules (see handout).
- Have students dress up in protective equipment.

Closure

(2–3 minutes)
- Restate the objectives in question form.
- Check students' knowledge and understanding of the concepts presented.
- If time permits, address any other questions the students may have.

Lesson plan / SAFETY

GRADE LEVEL _____ ROOM _____

SCHOOL _____ TEACHER _____

TIME REQUIRED (30 MINUTES) _____

Preparation in Classroom _____
_____
_____
_____
_____
_____

Anticipatory Planning _____
_____
_____
_____
_____
_____
_____
_____

Review of Previous Objectives: _____
_____
_____
_____
_____
_____

Three Specific Objectives:

1. _____
_____

2. _____
_____

3. _____
_____

Information to Be Presented Will Include:

(Topics) _____

_____

_____

_____

_____

_____

(Methods) _____

_____

_____

_____

_____

_____

(Lecture, demonstration, visual aids, group discussion) _____

_____

_____

_____

_____

_____

Guided Practice Activities _____

_____

_____

_____

_____

_____

Closure _____

_____

_____

_____

_____

_____

_____

NAME _____

List the items that would be in your Dental Emergency Kit.

1. _____

2. _____

3. _____

4. _____

5. _____

6. _____

7. _____

8. _____

9. _____

10. _____

11. _____

12. _____

NAME _____

List the safety rules that you will follow.

1. _____
2. _____
3. _____
4. _____
5. _____
6. _____
7. _____
8. _____
9. _____
10. _____
11. _____
12. _____

Repeat this statement for each safety rule listed above:

I will follow Rule No._____at all times.

Play Safe

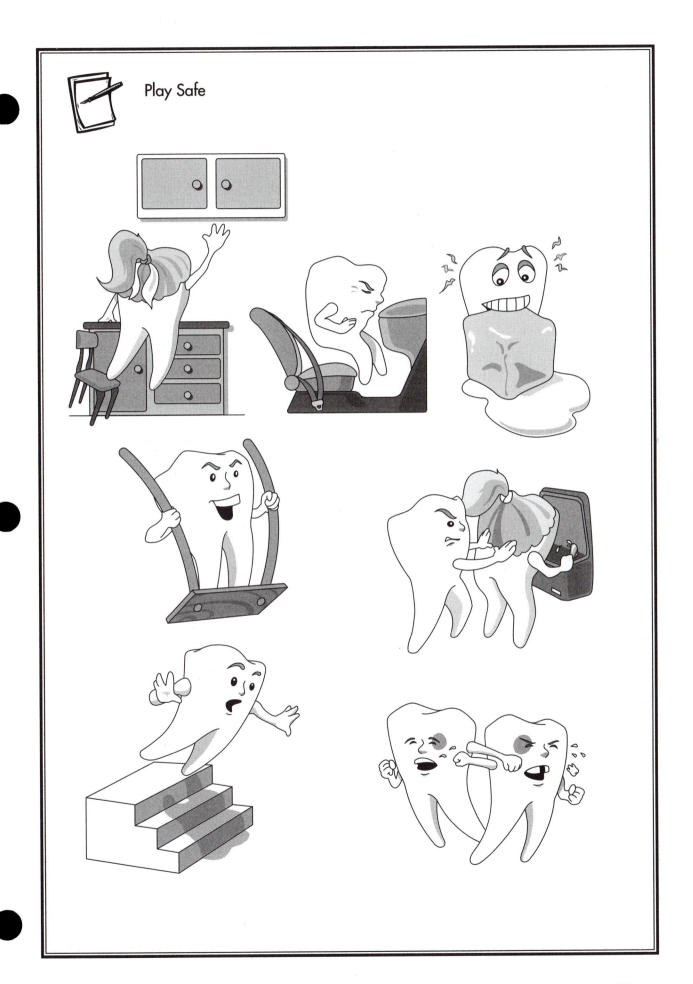

FIGURE 2–8   Play Safe   87

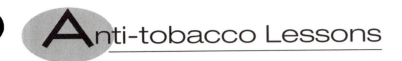

Anti-tobacco Lessons

Warning: Check with the school administration for specific protocols if you plan to bring any tobacco products onto school grounds.

Preparation

(5 minutes before beginning lesson) Display different forms of tobacco and tobacco products: cigarettes, cigars, pipe tobacco, smokeless tobacco (snuff, chewing tobacco).

Anticipatory Planning

(5 minutes)
- Review the previous lesson, if applicable.
- Introduce presenters.
- Describe the goals of today's lesson, the format of information, and general topics to be covered.
- Review classroom rules (K–3), if applicable.
- Survey the class' tobacco exposure or awareness. (Ask: "How many of you know of someone who uses smokeless tobacco or any form of tobacco?")

General Objectives by Grade Level

State specifically no more than three objectives appropriate for the classroom learning level that indicate what the majority of the students will be able to achieve by the completion of the lesson. Keep in mind that for every grade level you advance, the previous grade level objectives could also be used.

(2–3 minutes) Upon completion of this lesson, the student will be able to:

GR	OBJECTIVE
K	Distinguish between good and bad habits.
	Distinguish between good and bad air flow.
	Identify tobacco as a bad habit.
	Relate healthy lungs to breathing and air supply.
1	List three ways one can protect oneself from sidestream and secondary smoke.
2	Identify at least three parts of the body directly affected by tobacco use.
	Describe the possible effect of tobacco use on those parts.
3	Describe smokeless tobacco.
	Recognize smokeless tobacco as an unsafe alternative to cigarette smoking.
4	Define peer pressure.
	State at least three ways to say "no" to using tobacco.
	Identify at least two tricks used by advertisers to promote tobacco use.
5	Discuss social- and health-related consequences.
6	Include any or all of the above information.

Instruction/Information

(10 minutes) More than one topic may be included or combined with the guided practice segment (10 to 20 minutes). Use as many visuals as possible for grades K–3; group discussion may be more appropriate for grades 4–6.

- Discuss good habits versus bad habits.
- Show examples of or discuss the different types of tobacco.
- Use the handout illustrating Tobacco Tom's body structures to discuss the effects of tobacco.
- Discuss alternatives to tobacco, and alternatives to sidestream or second-hand smoke exposure.
- Present the fact sheet about tobacco (see appendix).
- Discuss the link between tobacco and oral cancers.
- Discuss social and health-related consequences of tobacco use.
- Present your survey of the cost of tobacco products.
- Relate the advertising tricks of the trade used by tobacco companies to entice new smokers.
- Review the most common concerns students have about tobacco use.

Good habits versus bad habits

Begin the discussion by defining the word "habit" (a tendency to do something over and over again, without really thinking about it). On the black/white board, list good habits at home and school, as follows:

- Brushing and flossing your teeth
- Combing your hair
- Washing your hands
- Eating healthy foods
- Playing safely
- Raising your hands
- Sitting quietly in your seats

Next, list bad habits at home and school, as follows:

- Putting objects in your mouth (erasers, pencils, pens, paper clips, pins, and coins)
- Talking out of turn
- Biting your nails
- Twisting your hair
- Smoking

Use visuals to reinforce the discussion. Have pictures of the following items:

- Good habits: (1) brushing, (2) flossing, (3) fluoride, (4) eating good foods, (5) good dental habits
- Bad habits: (1) dental decay; (2) sore, bleeding gums; (3) tobacco, tobacco plant, tobacco leaves, cigarettes, cigars, pipes, and smokeless tobacco; (4) stained teeth; (5) mouth sores; (6) unhealthy person

Use the following script to describe the good habit pictures you've provided and to discuss the benefits and consequences of their actions.

1. Brushing
   a. Benefit: Cleans teeth and gums and removes plaque so you have fewer cavities and less chance of bleeding gums.
   b. Consequence: Not brushing allows plaque to form on teeth, causing swollen gums and cavities.
2. Flossing
   a. Benefit: Removes plaque between teeth, helps prevent cavities, and keeps gums healthy.
   b. Consequence: Not flossing has the opposite effect.
3. Fluoride
   a. Benefit: Makes teeth hard and strong and helps prevent cavities.

   b. Consequence: Lack of fluoride leaves teeth without protection and more susceptible to decay.
  4. Eating good foods
   a. Benefit: Makes teeth and bodies healthy and strong.
   b. Consequence: Eating too many sugary or fatty foods increases acids, which attack the teeth causing cavities. It also builds fat in our bodies, making it harder for our hearts to work.
  5. Good dental habits
   a. Benefits: Good strong teeth and healthy bodies.
   b. Consequence: Tooth decay and gum disease.

Use the following script to describe the bad habit pictures:

1. Dental decay is a possible consequence of not brushing, flossing, or using fluorides.
2. Sore, bleeding gums are a consequence of not brushing and flossing.
3. The tobacco habit: Ask students, "Who knows where tobacco comes from?" (*Answer:* The tobacco plant.)
 a. Tobacco plant: Tobacco is grown in many parts of the United States as a crop, just like fruits and vegetables are grown by farmers.
 b. Tobacco leaves are cut and dried, then crushed until they look much like coffee grounds. They are then put into tobacco products to be sold.
 c. Cigarettes, cigars, and pipes are lit with a match so they will burn, causing smoke which is very dangerous to our bodies. The consequences of smoking include lung and heart disease.
 d. Smokeless tobacco is another kind of tobacco, also called snuff or chew, that is not lit but instead is put in the mouth between the cheek and gums. Using any form of tobacco is a bad habit because of the dangerous consequences.
4. Tobacco stains the teeth. Also, snuff and chew users have to spit, because if they swallowed the juices, it could hurt them and make them sick.
5. Tobacco gives us bad breath. It can also cause sores and white patches that turn into cancer. It can make our gums sore.
6. Unhealthy person: Tobacco can cause two serious diseases, lung cancer and heart disease, that harm our bodies and can make us very sick.

Tobacco Tom and the effects of tobacco

Make up a story about a boy named Tom. Talk about how his friends try to influence him to try a smoking tobacco product. Use pictures or make structures out of felt and display them on a flannel board to illustrate how tobacco affects different parts of the body: heart (enlarged), lungs (clogs the air sacs, making breathing more difficult), eyes (red and puffy), nose (irritated), teeth (yellow and stained). An additional unpleasant effect is the odor (smelly hair, breath, hands, clothes, environment).

This discussion can be followed by a guided practice activity in which students use the handout provided at the end of this lesson to illustrate the changes that occur with tobacco use.

Alternatives to smoking

Present the following healthy alternatives to smoking. Ask students if they can identify other healthy habits to replace smoking.

- Seek professional help from a dentist, dental hygienist, or physician about smoking cessation programs.
- Find a new—good—habit to replace smoking (e.g., eat carrots and other healthy snacks, chew sugarless gum).

Alternatives to sidestream or secondhand smoke exposure

Elicit from the class alternatives to staying in a smoke-filled room or other location by asking students what they would do if in that situation. Possible options include:

- Going into another room
- Going outside
- Asking the adult to please not smoke around you (explain that it makes it difficult for you to breathe, makes your eyes water, smells bad, etc.)
- Asking the smoker to go outside
- Rolling down the windows if in a car

Consequences of tobacco use

Discuss the following consequences that result from using tobacco products:

- Nicotine addiction (define addiction and explain that nicotine is a drug-like substance found in tobacco)
- Oral cancer
- Wearing down of tooth surface (chewing tobacco)
- Staining of teeth
- Increased salivation
- Bad breath
- Gum recession
- Tooth decay
- Dizziness
- Loss of smell and taste

Discussion: Smokeless tobacco fact sheet

Present the smokeless tobacco fact sheet (see appendix). Highlight the following points:

- A can of smokeless tobacco contains three times the amount of nicotine in one pack of cigarettes.
- Smokeless tobacco is a drug. It is as addicting as heroin or crack cocaine.
- A bug in a jar with a moistened tobacco leaf will die within a half hour from the toxins.
- The first time most people try smokeless tobacco, they get sick.
- The earlier the age at which a person first tries smokeless tobacco, the more likely he or she will become addicted.
- Within approximately 6 months of using smokeless tobacco, it is possible to recognize changes in the tissues of the mouth.
- The levels of bacteria in tobacco increase during the growth of the tobacco leaf, during processing, while it is on the shelf, and again in the mouth.

General Information: The Link Between Smokeless Tobacco and Oral Cancers

One estimate fixes the number of smokeless tobacco users in the United States at 22 million. Sales of smokeless tobaccos have increased by over 30 percent in the past 10 years, while sales of cigarettes, cigars, and pipe tobacco have declined. Industry analysts predict that the number of users could double over the next few years as health-conscious Americans look for alternatives to cigarette smoking.

Forms of smokeless tobacco include:

- Moist and dry snuff
- Loose-leaf chewing tobacco

- Plug or pressed-leaf chewing tobacco
- Fine-cut and twist chewing tobacco

Among the factors contributing to the growth in the numbers of smokeless tobacco users are the following:

- An increasing number of public places that forbid smoking
- Americans' increased participation in sports and outdoor activities in which participants need to keep their hands free
- The popularity of smokeless tobacco use among lifestyle and sports role models
- Weaning from cigarettes by former smokers
- The monetary savings of chewing tobacco compared with smoking cigarettes (a 3-ounce pouch of loose-leaf chewing tobacco can last a week)

Smokeless tobaccos, which tobacco manufacturers claim are a safe alternative to cigarette smoking, actually contain high concentrations of certain carcinogens (substances that cause cancer, as well as 30 metals and a radioactive compound called polonium-210) and create a dependence on nicotine, as do cigarettes. Constant contact with a wad of smokeless tobacco (called a "quid") can cause cancer of the esophagus, pharynx, larynx, stomach, and pancreas. Smokeless tobacco users are 50 times more likely to get oral cancer than non-users. These cancers can form within five years of regular use. Smokeless tobacco can also cause leukoplakia, a disease of the mouth characterized by white patches and oral lesions on the cheeks, gums, and/or tongue. Leukoplakia, which can lead to oral cancer, occurs in over half of all users in the first three years of use. Studies have found that 60 to 78 percent of smokeless tobacco users have oral lesions.

Nationwide, about 15,000 new cases of oral cancer are diagnosed each year, resulting in approximately 7,000 deaths. The incidence of oral cancer is almost three times higher in males than in females. Some signs of oral cancer include:

- Sores that fail to heal and bleed easily
- A lump or thickening
- Whitish patches
- Difficulty in chewing or swallowing food
- A sensation of something being caught in the throat

Other dangers of smokeless tobacco use include:

- Gum recession and increased sensitivity to heat and cold, resulting from exposed roots
- Drifting and loss of teeth caused by damage to gum tissue
- Abrasion of tooth enamel due to high levels of sand and grit contained in smokeless tobaccos
- Tooth discoloration and bad breath
- Tooth decay caused by varying levels of sugar added to smokeless tobacco to improve its taste
- Possible decreased athletic performance due to constriction of blood vessels caused by nicotine use

Discussion and group activity: Social and health-related consequences of tobacco use

Divide the class into groups. Give each group a health-related or social issue from those listed in Tables 2–10 and 2–11. Have each group discuss the issue and then present their views to the rest of the class.

Table 2–10   Health-Related Consequences of Tobacco Use

Not Smoking Cigarettes	*Smoking Cigarettes*
Better health	Lung cancer
Able to taste food	Lung diseases
Able to smell	Cough
Breathe easily	Shortness of breath
More energy	Loss of stamina
Won't get addicted	More frequent illness
Greater endurance	Heart disease
	Addiction
	Dizziness
	Nausea
	Deadened taste buds/smell
Not Using Smokeless Tobacco	*Using Smokeless Tobacco*
Better sense of taste	Gum disease
Better sense of smell	Cancer of the mouth
Healthier gums	Cancer of the larynx
Fewer cavities	Decreased athletic performance
Won't develop a habit	Loss of teeth
	Addiction
	Tooth decay

Table 2–11   Social Consequences of Tobacco Use

Not Smoking Cigarettes	*Smoking Cigarettes*
Save money	Empty wallet
Better reputation	Changing group of friends
Won't pollute the air	Bad breath
Won't fit with certain groups	Yellow teeth
More attractive	Smelly clothes
Cleaner body	Get in trouble
No stains on teeth	Cause fires
No odors	Get wrinkles earlier
Greater personal control	Holes in clothes
Serve as an example to others	Offend people
Not Using Smokeless Tobacco	*Using Smokeless Tobacco*
Save money	Empty wallet
Won't spit	Spit a lot
Won't have bad breath	Bad breath
Clean teeth	Yellow teeth
More attractive	Leaves stuck to teeth and gums

Computing the cost of tobacco products

Survey the price of tobacco products in a local store. Write on the black/white board the cost for a pack of cigarettes (approximately $2.99 a pack per day). Then write the following equations:

2 packs a day @ $2.99 = $5.98 × 7 days a week = $41.86 × 32 weeks per year = $1339.52

Advertising tricks of the trade

Following is a list of some common advertising claims or associations that are used to lure new smokers. Bring in ads from magazines to illustrate as many of these techniques as possible. Ask students to identify what "tricks" are being used to sell the product in each picture.

- "Amazing new product (or invention)": Stating that their brand is new and therefore better or more effective than others
- Comparison: Comparing their "superior" brand to another "inferior" brand
- Health appeal: Suggesting that their brand can do wonders for health
- Sex appeal: Using beautiful women or handsome men to sell their brand
- Symbols: Emphasizing a brand's logo or catchy saying
- Bandwagon: Claiming that "everybody" is using their product and making you feel left out if you don't use it, too
- Having fun: Showing people having fun and implying that using their brand will help people enjoy themselves more
- Mockery or put-down: Leading people to feel that they are doing something wrong or have failed if they don't use certain brands
- Snob appeal: Claiming that rich people use their brand or saying that even though their brand costs more, it's worth it
- Testimonial: Showing a famous person using a certain brand or talking about how wonderful a particular brand is

Students' most common concerns

Recite the following questions and concerns to the class, and ask if they have ever wondered about them. Follow each question or concern with the response indicated. Students may wish to address other questions or concerns, as well. Be sure to involve the whole class and address everyone's concerns.

CONCERN: "My little league coach uses smokeless tobacco and he's healthy (and older, wiser, my idol, etc.)."

Response: Explain that it is probably a habit with him. He may even be addicted. Review the meanings of these terms. Make the habit or the addiction the bad guy—not the person.

CONCERN: "Will my brother die if he keeps using smokeless tobacco?"

Response: Try to avoid using the word "die." The phrase "very sick" is better, but if you have to use the expression, say, "Many people who use smokeless tobacco don't die, especially if they stop using it. But, yes, some people do die."

CONCERN: "My mother smokes. I don't want anything to happen to her."

Response: Again, focus on the habit, not the person. Focus on how she will be getting healthier if she stops, not on the possibility of dying.

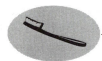

(10 minutes)

Guided Practice Activities

This segment may be combined with the preceding instruction/information segment. Visual aids are included at the end of the lesson.

- Have students complete the good habits versus bad habits matching exercise (see handout).
- Have students label Tobacco Tom's body structures and show how they are affected by tobacco use (see handout).
- Play the LUNGO game.
- Present the peer pressure group activity.
- Review various types of tobacco products, if displayed during the anticipatory or instruction/information segments of this lesson.

LUNGO GAME

Use the LUNGO card handout at the end of this lesson to keep score. Write out several questions and statements (true/false, multiple choice, fill in) regarding tobacco on individual cards. Or, have students brainstorm the questions that will be asked. Number the questions as follows: L1 through L5, U1 through U5, N1 through N5, G1 through G5, O1 through O5.

Have each student draw a question from the numbered cards. If the question is correct, the student blocks out or colors in the square on the score card that corresponds to the question number. The goal is to spell the word LUNGO by having five spaces in the same line blocked out horizontally, or to block all of the squares vertically.

Table 2–12   Peer Pressure Group Activity: What Would You Do?

Group 1

Some friends form a new club and in order to become a member, you must smoke a full cigarette.

Group 2

While sitting with a group of friends, the school's bully approaches and offers you a cigarette.

Group 3

You are at a friend's house watching TV and both parents are smoking continuously. It is making your eyes water and you feel very uncomfortable.

Group 4

At a ballgame, someone puts a wad of smokeless tobacco in his mouth and passes the package on to you.

Group 5

You are sitting in a restaurant enjoying your meal when a person at the next table lights up a cigarette. Thick smoke is blowing into your face and stopping you from enjoying your food.

Group 6

Your older brother or sister has just picked up a new habit of smoking and thinks it is very cool. He or she wants you to join in this new habit.

The game ends when the first student achieves this goal. For an even greater challenge, have the students play until all the spaces are blocked out. Students can participate as individuals or teams.

PEER PRESSURE GROUP ACTIVITY

Divide the class up into six groups. Assign each group a situation from those listed in Table 2–12. Have each group discuss how they would respond to the situation. Share the answers and comments with the rest of the class.

Closure

(2–3 minutes)

- Restate the objectives in question form.
- Check students' knowledge and understanding of the concepts presented.
- If time permits, address any other questions the students may have.

This information is summarized from CATS (Children Against Tobacco) workshop sponsored through The Dental Health Foundation, Mary Maurer, M.Ed., Tobacco Education, 1991.

Leſſon plɑn / ANTI-TOBACCO

GRADE LEVEL _____ ROOM _____

SCHOOL _____ TEACHER _____

TIME REQUIRED (30 MINUTES) _____

Preparation in Classroom _____

_____

_____

_____

_____

_____

Anticipatory Planning _____

_____

_____

_____

_____

_____

_____

_____

_____

Review of Previous Objectives: _____

_____

_____

_____

_____

_____

_____

Three Specific Objectives:

1. _____

_____

2. _____

_____

3. _____

_____

Information to Be Presented Will Include:

(Topics) _____

_____

_____

_____

_____

_____

(Methods) _____

_____

_____

_____

_____

_____

(Lecture, demonstration, visual aids, group discussion) _____

_____

_____

_____

_____

_____

Guided Practice Activities _____

_____

_____

_____

_____

Closure _____

_____

_____

_____

_____

_____

_____

Draw a line from a good or bad habit to its consequence.

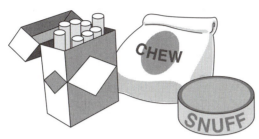

Using tobacco

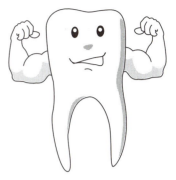

Happy tooth

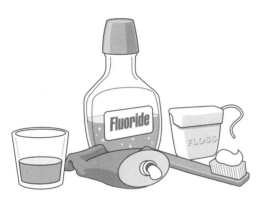

Brushing and flossing

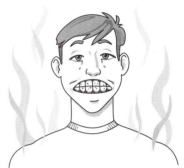

Very sick

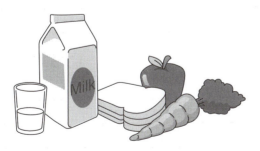

Eating healthy foods

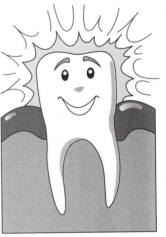

Fewer cavities and
healthy gums

NAME _____

Draw a line to connect the words next to Tobacco Tom with the correct body parts.

Draw in the changes that occur in Tom's body when using tobacco.

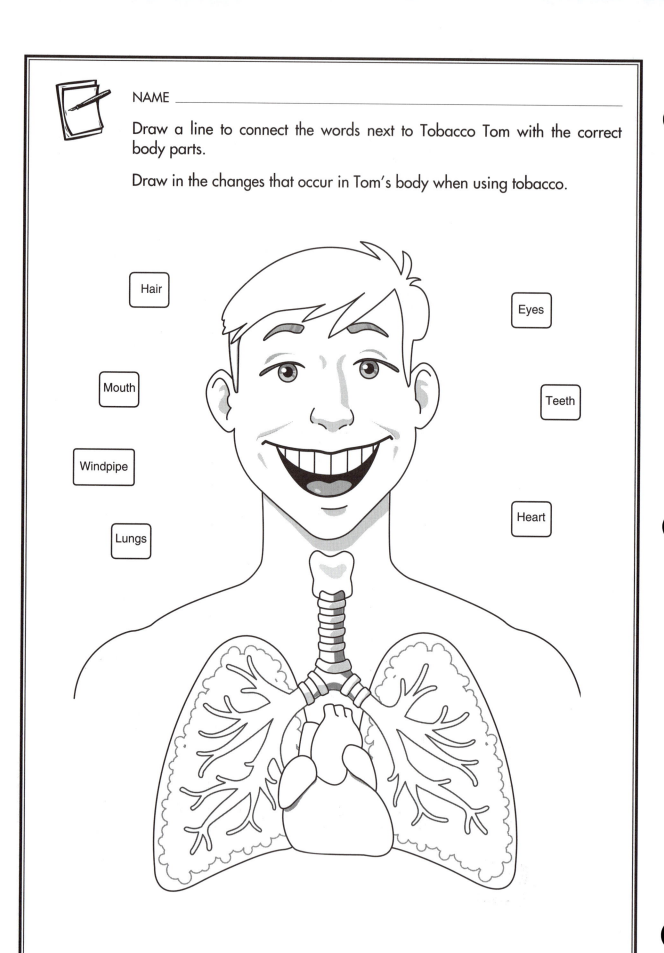

102

LUNGO Game

	L	U	N	G	O
1.					
2.					
3.					
4.					
5.					

he Dental Office Visit

Preparation

(5 minutes before beginning lesson) Dress up as a member of the dental health team; post large charts listing all the names and functions of the dental health team members; bring infection control gear; assemble the following items: a large tooth model and brush, tray of instruments, extracted teeth with fillings, sealants, and so on.

Anticipatory Planning

(5 minutes)
- Review the previous lesson, if applicable.
- Introduce presenters.
- Describe the goals of today's lesson, the format of information, and general topics to be covered.
- Review classroom rules (K–3), if applicable.
- Survey the class about a few of their recent dental office experiences.

General Objectives by Grade Level

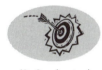

(2–3 minutes)

State specifically no more than three objectives appropriate for the classroom learning level that indicate what the majority of the students will be able to achieve by the completion of the lesson. Keep in mind that for every grade level you advance, the previous grade level objectives could also be used.

Upon completion of this lesson, the student will be able to:

GR	OBJECTIVE
K	Identify the importance of our teeth.
	Identify the members of the dental health team.
1	Describe instruments and equipment used in a dental office.
	Describe infection control procedures.
	Identify various duties of the dental health team in the dental office.
	Explain the function of a dental sealant.
2	Name and describe the functions of our teeth.
3	Relate the history of dentistry to modern times.
	Develop an appreciation for modern dental practice and procedures.
4	Include any or all of the above information.
5	Include any or all of the above information.
6	Include any or all of the above information.

Instruction/Information

(10 minutes) More than one topic may be included or combined with the guided practice segment (10 to 20 minutes). Use as many visual aids as possible for grades K–3; group discussion may be more appropriate for grades 4–6.

- Discuss the importance of teeth.
- Present the history of dentistry and review questions.

- Describe the members of the dental health team and outline their various duties in the dental office.
- Describe the instruments used in a dental office.
- Explain the importance of infection control during dental procedures.
- Discuss the use of sealants.
- Show diagrams of orthodontia problems and discuss their correction.

Importance of teeth

Present Figures 2–9 and 2–10. Describe the parts of the tooth and the functions of teeth. Explain that teeth are used for:

- *Eating.* As we chew, our teeth help us cut, tear, and grind the food into small pieces. As the food is broken down, it is also mixed with saliva and the first phase of digestion is begun. If food is swallowed without being properly chewed, the stomach has to work harder and longer to digest it. This may give us a stomachache.
- *Talking.* Verbal: As air comes from our throat, it is caught with our lips, our teeth, and our tongue. In this way sound becomes word forms. Non-verbal: The positions of the lips, teeth, and jaws also play an important role in making expressions.
- *Appearance.* Teeth help to form the face. Without teeth, the mouth sinks in and looks funny. Clean teeth give us a pretty smile.

Next, list the names and functions of the different types of teeth:

- Incisors: The four upper and four lower front teeth. The four central incisor are in the very front; the four lateral incisors are next to them. The incisors are used to cut food. They are included in both adult and primary dentition.
- Cuspid: The two upper and two lower corner teeth. The cuspids are used to tear food. They are included in both adult and primary dentition.
- Bicuspids: The four upper and four lower teeth next to the cuspids. The bicuspids crush and tear food. They are included in the adult dentition.
- Molars: The upper and lower teeth that make up the rest of the dentition. The molars are used to grind food. In the adult dentition, there are 12 molars; in the primary dentition, 8 (the first and second premolars are replaced with the adult bicuspids).

Describe the parts of the tooth:

- Crown: The top portion of the tooth that is seen in the mouth.
- Root(s): The bottom portion of the tooth that holds the tooth in place. The incisors have one root; the bicuspids, one of two roots; the cuspids, one root; and the molars, two roots on the lower teeth and three roots on the upper teeth.

Review the tooth tissues and supporting structures identified in Figure 2–9 (enamel, dentin, cementum, pulp, alveolar bone, lamina dura, periodontal ligament, and apex). This review can also be combined with the guided practice activity later in this lesson.

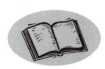

**Story of
Dentistry**

The History of Dentistry

No one knows who the first dentist was or when he or she lived. It may be that the first dentist was a friend of someone who was troubled by a toothache, and that this person helped cure the pain by using a primitive chisel to knock out the tooth. For thousands of years, people blamed toothaches on evil spirits, so the first dentist may have been a medicine man or woman who practiced magic or the tribal religious leader.

Eventually, people began searching for something other than magic to relieve a toothache. They started experimenting with various materials and substances that they hoped would bring them relief. They tried herbs and offensive smells, which were usually aimed at driving evil spirits out. (Bad-smelling mixtures were thought to offend the evil spirits, thereby driving them out of the aching tooth.)

Dental knowledge has evolved slowly. It has taken thousands of years to reach the point we are at today. Here's how a dentist might have treated you if you had lived 250, 500, 1000, or even 3000 years ago.

- An Egyptian dentist might have advised a patient to treat a toothache by splitting a mouse in half and rubbing it over the aching tooth.
- A Greek dentist living in the 5th century BC would have used a mouse in a prescription for curing bad breath.
- A dentist living during the Middle Ages would have tried curing a toothache by having the patient inhale smoke. This is because dentists at the time were convinced that a toothache was caused by worms that got into the tooth. Thus, it was thought that fumigating the teeth with smoke would kill the worms.
- The early Chinese used arsenic to cure a toothache. It worked to a degree, because it killed the pulp of the tooth. But the surrounding tissue would usually be damaged, which led to an abscessed tooth. As late as 1850, dentists in the United States also used arsenic to kill the pulp before they extracted a tooth.

Aristotle, a famous Greek philosopher who lived in the 3rd century BC, was one of the earliest people to associate sweets with tooth decay. "Figs and soft sweets," he said, "produced damage to the teeth, because small particles adhere between the teeth where they easily become the cause of putrefactive processes."

The Etruscans, who lived in central Italy from 1000 BC to 400 BC, were the most advanced of all the ancients in the act of mechanical dentistry. They were very advanced in making crowns, bridges, and false teeth.

Roman aristocrats practiced restorative dentistry for esthetic rather than health reasons. They were interested in having false teeth to improve their appearance rather than as an aid to digestion.

Dentistry during the Middle Ages moved backward from where it had been during the Roman and Etruscan times. Barber-surgeons became recognized as persons with the skill to shave a man's face, cut his hair, extract his teeth, and perform minor surgery.

The Plymouth Colony brought the first dentist to North America about 20 years after the first Pilgrims arrived in 1620. His name was W. Dinley, and shortly after his arrival, he perished in a snowstorm as he was traveling to Roxbury to pull a tooth for a patient.

In April, 1768, Dr. John Baker, the first competent dentist to practice in the American colonies, left Boston and went to New York. His advertisement in the *New York Journal* claimed that he could cure scurvy, fill hollow teeth with lead or gold, and make false teeth that looked as good as a person's natural teeth. (False teeth at that time were made from ivory, and they neither fit well nor looked as nice as natural teeth.)

One of our most famous Revolutionary War heroes, Paul Revere, was a dentist. The most famous false teeth in American history were those worn by our first president, George Washington. He had several sets of false teeth, but none were made from wood; rather, all were made from ivory.

The world's first dental school opened its doors in 1840 in Baltimore, Maryland. Until then, dentists got their training through an apprenticeship program, supplemented with whatever dental books were available. They had no background or knowledge of anatomy, pathology, or other related sciences. It took many years for the idea of a dental school to take hold. The changes in dental education were slow and gradual, but eventually the profession realized that a higher quality of training could be attained at a dental college rather than through an apprenticeship program.

Today, all dentists must graduate from a dental college, then pass a state licensing examination before they can practice dentistry. This is one reason that history's most highly trained and capable dentists are practicing today. They are doing things that the dentists of the past could only dream about. They can treat and cure gum disease, straighten crooked teeth, and aid in the prevention of dental disease.

Follow-up Discussion: The History of Dentistry

Have students address the following points as a follow-up to the story:

- Describe what it would be like to go to a dentist who lived 150 years ago.
- Are we caring for our teeth today in ways that people living 50 to 100 years from now will find strange?
- For the first time in history, we can prevent dental disease. Explain how.

Members of the dental health team

Describe each of the members of the dental health team and explain their roles:

- Dentist (DDS or DMD): A licensed professional who examines the teeth for decay; prepares and fills the teeth with sealants, fillings, crowns, bridges, partials, or dentures; and performs extractions and localized surgery. A dentist may clean the teeth or delegate this to a registered or licensed dental hygienist.
- Registered or Licensed Dental Hygienist (RDH/LDH): A licensed professional who examines the teeth for decay; cleans and polishes the teeth; takes and processes the radiographs (x-ray pictures); applies fluoride and sealants to protect the teeth; gives oral hygiene instructions; and provides nutritional counseling. The RDH/LDH may also sterilize the instruments. (Note: Duties may vary in each state.)
- Registered Dental Assistant (RDA): A licensed professional who assists the dentist, hygienists, or front office personnel before, after, or during the dental procedure. Like the RDH/LDH, the RDA may take and process the radiographs, give oral hygiene instructions, provide nutritional counseling, polish the teeth, and apply fluoride. The registered dental assistant may also be responsible for sterilizing the instruments. (Note: Duties may vary in each state.)
- Dental Assistant (DA): A professional who assists the dentist, hygienists, or front office personnel before, after, or during the dental procedure. The DA may take and process the radiographs, give oral hygiene instructions, and provide nutritional counseling. The DA may also sterilize the instruments. Some assistants are specially trained and licensed to work in various dental speciality offices (described below). (Note: Duties may vary in each state.)
- Front office person: A professional who greets the patients, assists them in making appointments, handles billing and insurance forms, and processes information into the computer. This person may also assist with the dental procedures as needed.
- Dental Laboratory Technician (DLT): A professional specially trained to make the crowns, bridges, partials, and dentures for patients in a dental office. Some dental laboratory technicians work in a dental office; others have their own separate offices.

Discuss the different types of dental specialty offices:

- Dental Public Health: The branch of dentistry that deals with the community and public health of dentistry as its practice
- Endodontics: The branch of dentistry concerned with diagnosis, treatment, and prevention of diseases of the dental pulp and its surrounding tissues
- Oral/Maxillofacial Surgeon: The branch of dentistry that deals with extraction and reconstruction of the jaw
- Orthodontics: The branch of dentistry that deals with prevention and correction of irregularities of the teeth
- Pedodontics: The branch of dentistry that deals with the care of children's teeth
- Periodontics: The branch of dentistry that deals with the treatment of diseases of the tissues surrounding the teeth
- Prosthodontics: The branch of dentistry that deals with the construction, making, and fitting of artificial teeth

Dental instruments

Bring in several of the instruments used in a dental office (mounting them on a tray for visibility). Explain the use of each instrument.

- Mouth mirror: Used to see the teeth
- Explorer: Used to count the teeth
- Curet/scaler: A small pick used to clean teeth
- Prophy-angle/cup: Used to polish teeth
- Vacuum tip: Used to remove excess water from the mouth
- Fluoride tray: Used to put fluoride on the teeth

Discuss the other equipment that patients would find: an x-ray machine, lead apron, air–water syringe, dental chair, and handpiece.

Infection control

Dress up with all the protective OSHA (Occupational Safety and Health Administration) gear and ask the class, "Why do we wear this in the dental office?" (*Answer:* To prevent the spread of germs from one person to another.) Discuss the importance of washing your hands before eating, after using the toilet, and so on to remove any germs. Define "germs." Explain that several steps are taken in the dental office to protect the dental office personnel and the patient from catching any germs. Protective gear includes:

- Eye wear: To protect our eyes from splatter
- Mask: To protect our mouth and nose
- Long gowns: To protect our bodies
- Gloves: To protect our hands

Explain that barriers are placed over the dental operatory (the chair, light, handpiece, etc.) to protect us from germs, and that sterilizers are used to kill the germs on dental instruments.

Sealants

Discuss how sealants are used to protect children's teeth from cavities. Explain that sealants are a clear or opaque coating that goes over the top (occlusal) portion of the back teeth (molars). They are applied to the teeth to keep the germs (plaque) from entering into the top of the molars through the grooves in the tooth surface. Sealants are applied when the molars first erupt in a child's mouth (at about 6 and 11 years of age) to give maximum protection. They are not placed in adults, only in children.

Orthodontia problems

Refer to Figure 2–11, which illustrates three common orthodontia problems: crowded teeth, overbite, and crossbite. Discuss the following problems associated with misaligned teeth:

- Cause problems with speaking
- Interfere with chewing and, therefore, lead to improper food selection
- Put a strain on the jaws and muscles leading to jaw pain
- Cause facial deformities leading to emotional and psychological problems
- Make it difficult to brush and floss, especially when teeth are tightly spaced
- Allow plaque to accumulate, leading to tooth decay, gum disease, and bone loss
- Lead to a poor self-image

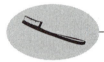

(10 minutes)

Guided Practice Activities

This segment may be combined with the preceding instruction/information segment. Visual aids are included at the end of the lesson.

- Present the story of how Mary and Mikey Molar get sealants.
- Relate the play or story: Timmy Visits the Dentist.
- Have students identify the tooth structures (see handout).
- Present the comparisons of animal teeth.
- Many books are available about the visit to the dentist; provide a list to students (see Section Four).

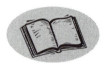

Mary and Mikey Molar Story

Mary and Mikey Molar Get Sealants

Create your own visuals to accompany this story, describing the procedure for applying a sealant.

Mary and Mikey are two molars that have just erupted. The tops (chewing surface) of Mary and Mikey Molar are very groovy. The two molars are worried about getting germs that can turn into decay. *(Check students' knowledge of the meaning of the word "decay.")* Mary and Mikey visit the dentist, who tells them that the dentist or the dental hygienist can put a special coating on the grooves that will prevent germs *(seal out the decay)* from getting into the tooth. Mary and Mikey think this is a good idea.

First Mary sits down in the dental chair. She sees the hose for water and for air. Mary's top enamel is brushed and cleaned with a small electric brushing machine. Next comes a liquid that has a bitter taste (like lemons). With a dab of cotton, the liquid is put around the molar. After a minute, there's a water spray. Mary needs to be very dry before the sealant can be applied. Once the sealant has been applied, a bright light may be placed over the tooth to help it dry. When the procedure is over, the top of Mary's tooth feels nice and smooth. Then it's Mikey's turn to get his sealant.

When Mary and Mikey leave the dentist's office, they are happy. They know that now they have sealants that will protect their tops (chewing surface).

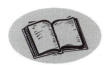

Timmy Visits the Dentist Play/Story

Timmy Visits the Dentist

The goals of this activity are to encourage children to ask their school nurse for help if they are in pain, to acquaint them with the personnel in the dental office, and to familiarize them with dental procedures.

Place chairs in the front of the room for each of the characters to sit on.

Actors and Props
Timmy: A notebook, book bag, backpack, or lunch box
Teacher: A ruler, chalk, or pointer
School Nurse: Red Cross arm badge
Timmy's Father: Necktie
Receptionist: Phone, magazine (for Timmy's father)
Assistant: Lab coat, bib clip, bib, tray of instruments, prophy
    cup, paste, fluoride tray, gauze, saliva ejector
Dentist: White shirt, gloves, mask, x-ray film in pocket
Hygienist: Lab coat, mask, gloves, Typodont (large tooth
    model), brush

After the actors are chosen and dressed appropriately, explain the reason for the masks and gloves (to avoid sharing germs). *Encourage the actors to do a little speaking during the reading of the story.*

Once upon a time there was a boy named Timmy who was a student at _____ school. *(Fill in appropriate name.)* His teacher was named Mr. Gonzales. One day, as Mr. Gonzales was about to put the spelling words on the board, he noticed Timmy sitting in the front row looking very, very sad. He asked Timmy what was wrong, and Timmy said he had a terrible toothache.

Mr. Gonzales sent Timmy to the school nurse. The nurse took a look at Timmy's tooth and told him he needed to go to the dentist. When she called Timmy's father, he explained that the family had no dentist and they did not have a lot of money, nor did they have a car to drive to a dental office. The nurse offered to try to find a dentist in their neighborhood that they could walk to and one that would let them pay some money each month until the bill was paid. The nurse gave Timmy's father a number to call.

Timmy's father called the dentist, and the receptionist said to come right in. Timmy's father picked him up at school and they walked to the dental office. At the office, the receptionist asked Timmy's father to sit in the waiting room and she gave him some forms to fill out and a magazine to read.

Soon the assistant came out to the waiting room and called Timmy's name. She took him into the operatory and put a bib on him. Next, she took an x-ray of the painful tooth. She went into a dark room to develop the x-ray, which she gave to the dentist. Then she took Timmy into the dentist's operatory.

The dentist checked Timmy's tooth and looked at the x-ray. Next, he put the tooth to sleep, removed the decay, and put a silver filling in the tooth. Afterward, the assistant took Timmy into the dental hygienist's room, where she cleaned his teeth using a tray of some special instruments, polished the teeth, and put fluoride on them. The dental hygienist reviewed toothbrushing and flossing instructions with Timmy.

At the end of the visit, as Timmy and his father left the dental office, the receptionist told Timmy to come back in 6 months for a checkup and teeth cleaning.

Follow-up Activities: Timmy Visits the Dentist

- Have students describe the duties of the dentist, receptionist, assistant, and hygienist.
- Have students name at least three instruments used in the dental office.

TOOTH STRUCTURES

Refer to Figure 2–9, which identifies the major tooth tissues and supporting structures. (Note: Each structure on the list that follows is keyed to the illustration by letter; e.g., A = enamel; B = dentin, etc.) Describe each part of the tooth to the class:

(A) Enamel: The tissue that covers the crown portion of the tooth. Enamel is the hardest substance in our body.

(B) Dentin: The tissue that makes up the bulk of the tooth structure.

(C) Cementum: The tissue that covers the root of the tooth.

(D) Pulp: The soft tissue that contains the blood, lymph, and nerves of the tooth.

(E) Alveolar bone: The bone that supports (holds) the teeth in the tooth socket.

(F) Lamina dura: The thin bone that lines the tooth socket.

(G) Periodontal ligament: The tissue that holds the tooth to the socket.

(H) Apex: The area at the end of the tooth root.

This illustration can also be reproduced as a handout for students to label and/or color.

ANIMAL TEETH COMPARISONS

If possible, bring in actual teeth to illustrate the differences between animal and human teeth. Or, bring pictures of as many different types of teeth (human or animal) as possible. Use diagrams to show how the shapes of various animals' teeth differ from human teeth.

Possible Activities

- Compare the size, shape, number, and function of each animal's teeth to the human teeth. Discuss how they vary and how they are similar.
- Discuss what devices we use to do some things that animals do with their teeth (e.g., squirrel uses his teeth to crack nuts, we use a nutcracker).
- Discuss why humans' teeth are more likely to be decayed than animals, the major factor being the type of food that is eaten. (Humans eat a lot of sweet foods.)
- Show pictures of animals as you discuss their teeth or have the children draw the animal pictures.

Preliminary Discussion

Teeth are shaped and formed according to their function. We use our teeth for eating, talking, and appearance, whereas animals' teeth are generally used for eating, obtaining food, and protection. Let's look at several different kinds of teeth.

Human Teeth

Humans have two sets of teeth: 20 primary (baby) and 32 permanent (adult) teeth. The teeth have four different shapes, and they vary in size and shape according to their use. The front teeth (incisors) cut, the pointed side teeth (cuspids) tear, the flat side teeth (bicuspids) crush, and the back teeth (molars) grind. (Refer to Fig. 2–10.)

Animal Teeth

Present several different examples from the following list:

- *Bird:* The bird has no teeth and cannot chew its food. Therefore, nature has made it so the bird can swallow its food whole. When the bird swallows its food, the unchewed food goes to a sort of storage tank called the crop. As the bird needs nourishment, the food passes from the crop to its stomach, which is called the gizzard. In the gizzard are pieces of gravel that the bird has swallowed on purpose. The gravel helps grind the food into tiny pieces so the bird's body can use it to be healthy. While this system works fine for the bird, we must chew our food well before swallowing it.

- *Beaver:* The beaver has four front teeth, two on top and two on the bottom. They are very strong and sharp. These teeth grow about 4 feet each year. However, they never look very long because they are continuously worn away. The beaver uses its teeth to cut down trees, which it uses to build a dam. Then, in the pond behind the dam, the beaver builds its home. The beaver's dam helps it catch food and hide from its enemies.
- *Elephant:* The elephant has two big front teeth that come out of its mouth. These teeth are called tusks. They weigh from 55 to 200 pounds and can be as long as 10 feet. The tusks are made of ivory, and the elephant uses them to eat and to fight its enemies.
- *Walrus:* The walrus also has two long front teeth called tusks that stick out of its mouth. Like the elephant's tusks, the walrus's are made of ivory. They are much smaller, though; usually between 14 and 26 inches long. The walrus uses its tusks to tear seaweed loose and to dig up clams to eat. They also help the walrus move along the ice and land, in much the same way that we use ski poles.
- *Whale:* Whales are the largest living mammals (warm-blooded animals that nurse their babies). Some kinds of whales have as many as 3000 teeth in each jaw. But they are only 1/8-inch long. Other whales have no teeth. Most whales eat very small fish and swallow them whole. Therefore, whales don't really need teeth.
- *Vampire bat:* The vampire bat has two upper front teeth that are triangular and project forward. The edges and tip are razor sharp, enabling the bat to cut into the skin of its victims and suck their blood, which it eats as food.
- *Squirrel:* The squirrel has very strong teeth. It uses its teeth to crack the shells of nuts so it can eat the nutmeats for food.
- *Snake:* The snake has many tiny sharp teeth that help it swallow its food. The snake's mouth can be stretched to several times its normal size in order to swallow large animals. Many poisonous snakes have two long upper front teeth, called fangs. They are used to bite and squirt poison into the snake's victims. These fangs are hidden under a flap of skin when the snake's mouth is closed.
- *Cow:* The cow has no upper front teeth, but in their places are horny pads. Therefore, the cow cannot use just its teeth to get food. To pull grass out of the ground, the cow must grip it between the bottom teeth and the upper horny pads and then jerk its head back. The cow's back teeth are very flat. This is because the cow chews its food all day long and wears the teeth down.
- *Dog:* The dog has 42 strong teeth, including 2 upper teeth called canine or eye teeth. These teeth are very sharp and pointed. The dog uses these teeth to fight its enemies and to tear meat into smaller pieces that it can eat.
- *Cat:* The cat has 29 to 30 teeth. It also has canine or eye teeth similar to those of the dog.
- *Ape:* The ape's teeth are the most similar to those of humans. Both the ape and the human have 32 teeth. However, the ape's jaw is longer, and it has two very pointed teeth in each jaw.

Closure

(2–3 minutes)

- Restate the objectives in question form.
- Check students' knowledge and understanding of the concepts presented.
- If time permits, address any other questions the students may have.

Le**ss**on pl**a**n / DENTAL OFFICE VISIT

GRADE LEVEL _____ ROOM _____

SCHOOL _____ TEACHER _____

TIME REQUIRED (30 MINUTES) _____

Preparation in Classroom _____

_____
_____
_____
_____
_____

Anticipatory Planning _____

_____
_____
_____
_____
_____
_____

Review of Previous Objectives: _____

_____
_____
_____
_____
_____

Three Specific Objectives:

1. _____

_____

2. _____

_____

3. _____

_____

Information to Be Presented Will Include:

(Topics) _____
_____
_____
_____
_____
_____

(Methods) _____
_____
_____
_____
_____
_____

(Lecture, demonstration, visual aids, group discussion) _____
_____
_____
_____
_____
_____

Guided Practice Activities _____
_____
_____
_____
_____

Closure _____
_____
_____
_____
_____
_____
_____

Tooth Tissues and Supporting Structures

Directions: Write the names of the parts of a tooth on the lines below.

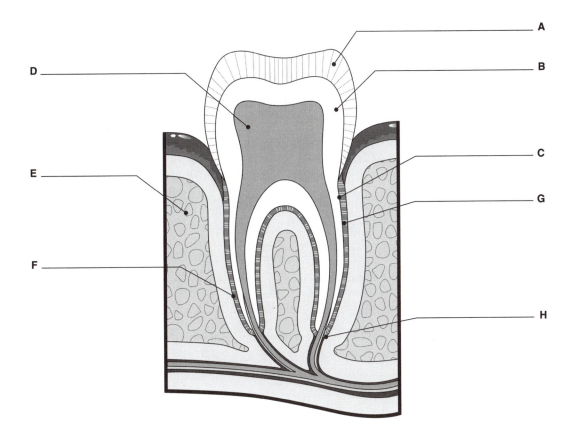

A. Enamel: the tissue that covers the crown portion of the tooth. Enamel is the hardest substance in our body.

B. Dentin: The tissue that makes up the bulk of the tooth structure.

C. Cementum: The tissue that covers the root of the tooth.

D. Pulp: the soft tissue which contains the blood, lymph, and nerve systems of the tooth.

E. Alveolar bone: The bone which supports (holds) the teeth in the tooth socket.

F. Lamina dura: Thin bone lining the tooth socket.

G. Periodontal ligament: The tissue which holds the tooth to the socket.

H. Apex: The area at the end of the tooth root.

FIGURE 2–9   Tooth Tissues and Supporting Structures   117

Types of Teeth

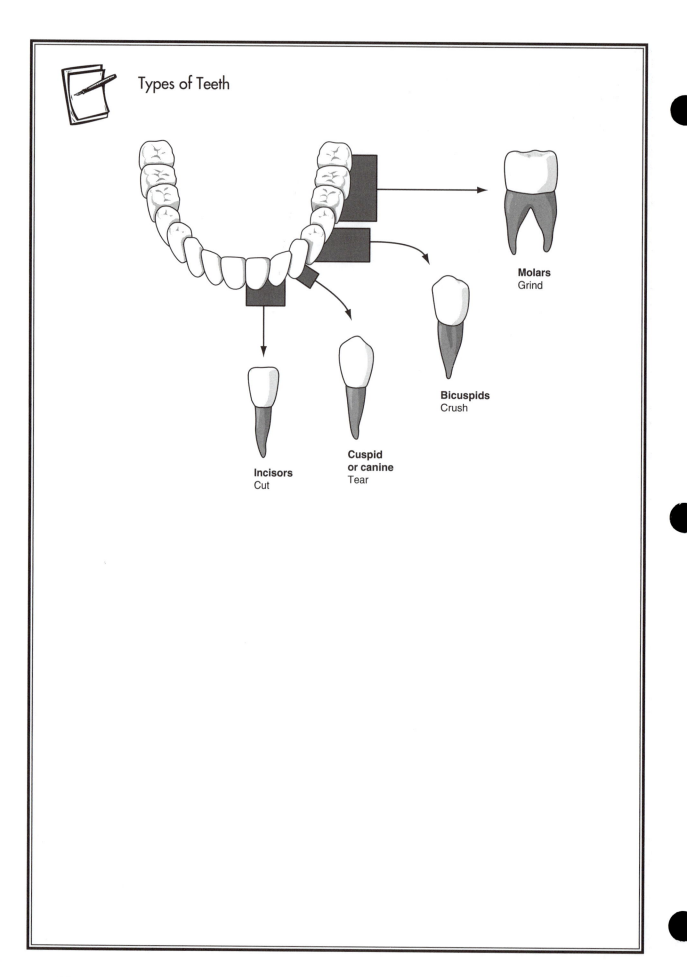

Incisors
Cut

Cuspid
or canine
Tear

Bicuspids
Crush

Molars
Grind

Orthodontic Problems and Consequences

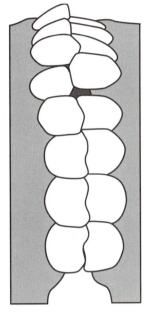

Crowded teeth: normal jaw

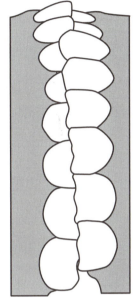

Crossbite: lower teeth in front of upper teeth

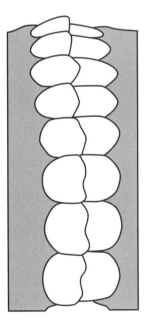

Proper occlusion, or bite

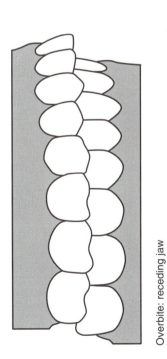

Overbite: receding jaw

FIGURE 2–11   Orthodontic Problems and Consequences.   119

Last Visit: Wrap Up and Review

Preparation

(5 minutes before beginning lesson)   Assemble a big tooth model, toothbrush, and other items needed for the lesson.

Anticipatory Planning

(5 minutes)
- Introduce presenters.
- Describe the goals of today's lesson, the format of information, and general topics to be covered.
- Review classroom rules (K–3), if applicable.

General Objectives by Grade Level

(2–3 minutes)   State specifically no more than three objectives appropriate for the classroom learning level that indicate what the majority of the students will be able to achieve by the completion of the lesson. Keep in mind that for every grade level you advance, the previous grade level objectives could also be used. In this lesson, take the opportunity to check for knowledge and restate a variety of objectives previously given to the class.

Upon completion of this lesson, the student will be able to perform the following objectives and respond appropriately for his or her grade level:

- Describe the process of dental disease and its consequences.
- State how to prevent dental disease by: toothbrushing, flossing, using fluoride, eating healthy snacks and food, eating sugar in moderation, using sealants, and visiting the dentist.

Instruction/Information

(10 minutes)   More than one topic may be included or combined with the guided practice segment (10 to 20 minutes). Use as many visuals as possible for grades K–3; group discussion may be more appropriate for grades 4–6.

- Review the information that has been given during the year.
- Present the typical review questions to test students' knowledge.

Review of information

Review the information presented in previous lessons with emphasis on the following areas:

- Plaque control
- Prevention of dental diseases
- Toothbrushing
- Flossing
- Fluoride use
- Nutrition
- Dental sealants
- Visiting the dentist

Typical review questions

The following review questions can be used to tests students' understanding of the information that has been presented throughout the year. They can also be used with the tooth-tac-toe, stop the pirates, and blackboard football games presented in the guided practice activities segment later in this lesson.

All Grade Levels

1. What is the sticky film that collects on our teeth after we've eaten food? (*Plaque.*)
2. How do you spell plaque? (*P-L-A-Q-U-E.*)
3. What does fluoride do for our teeth? (*It makes them strong.*)
4. How often should we brush our teeth? (*At least 2 times a day.*)
5. What happens if the plaque is not removed from your teeth? (*It forms an acid that can cause cavities or decay.*)
6. List two reasons why are teeth are important? (*Possible answers: They help us to eat, talk, and look nice.*)
7. Name two things we can do to keep our teeth forever. (*Possible answers: brush, floss, use fluoride, eat healthy foods.*)

Grades 2–3

1. Name three foods that are bad for our teeth.
2. How do we get plaque out from between our teeth where the toothbrush cannot reach? (*By flossing.*)
3. Name two drinks that would be good for our teeth.
4. Name two sources of fluoride.
5. Describe at least one safety rule.
6. Name two places where the plaque likes to hide.

Grades 4–6

1. Spell fluoride. (*F-L-U-O-R-I-D-E.*)
2. Name three sources of topical fluoride. (*Toothpaste, mouth rinse, fluoride trays at the dentist's office.*)
3. Name three sources of systemic fluoride. (*Possible answers: green leafy vegetables, fluoride tablets, fluoridated water, fish, tuna, fluoride drops.*)
4. Describe what you would do for a knocked-out tooth. (*Put it back in, put it in milk, or wrap it in gauze and see a dentist as soon as possible.*)
5. List two specifications for a good toothbrush. (*Soft bristles, right size for your mouth, straight narrow bristles not frayed or worn out.*)
6. Describe the dental disease process. (*Plaque + Sugar = Acid; Acid + Healthy tooth = Decay.*)

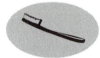

(10 minutes)   ## Guided Practice Activities

This segment may be combined with the preceding instruction/information segment. Visual aids are included at the end of the chapter.

- Present the melodrama for dental health: Trouble in Open Wide (grades K–6).
- Play the tooth-tac-toe game (grades K–6).
- Play the stop the pirates game (grades K–6).

- Have the students find five things that will keep their teeth healthy (grades K–3) (see handout).
- Give a quiz or post-test to check students' dental IQ (grades 2–6).
- Play the tooth sleuth game (grades 2–6).
- Play blackboard football (grades 3–6).

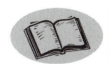

Trouble in
Open Wide
Melodrama

Trouble in Open Wide

Introduce the characters (see Fig. 2–12) and ask students in the class to give a specific response when each character is mentioned. For example, when you say Boss Plaque's name, the students should say, "Boo-hiss."

Choose four students to hold name cards. Each name card should have a character's name on one side and the appropriate response on the other. You may also want to draw big pictures of the characters on poster board (punch two holes at the top of the board tie string to wear over neck for the students to wear as a costume (refer to Fig. 2–12).

Characters
Cowboy Healthy Smile: (hero) "Wow"
Sheriff Smilin' Sam: (hero) "To the rescue"
Boss Plaque: (villain) "Boo-hiss"
Deputy Fluoride: (heroine) "Hurray"

Today we're going to participate in a melodrama called "Trouble in Open Wide." It's a toothful tale from the wild, Wild West.

Our story takes place in an old Wild West town called Open Wide. Open Wide is surrounded by the Lucky Lips mountains. In Open Wide there lived our hero, Cowboy Healthy Smile *(Flash card: Wow!)*. Now Cowboy Healthy Smile *(Flash card: Wow!)* was very useful, helping out at the Talk Shop. Cowboy Healthy Smile *(Flash card: Wow!)* was always eager to help say words and letters clearly. He loved to help with talking.

Cowboy Healthy Smile *(Flash card: Wow!)* also worked at the Eatin' Place. He was a very good muncher and cruncher. He was always ready to help out with eating. He also was happy to make a healthy smile. Why sometimes, Cowboy Healthy Smile *(Flash card: Wow!)* was so busy, he had to help with all three—talking, eating, and smiling at the same time!

One day our villain, Boss Plaque *(Flash card: Boo-hiss)* crept into Open Wide on his icky-sticky feet. He had every intention of taking over the town and capturing Cowboy Healthy Smile *(Flash card: Wow!)*. Boss Plaque *(Flash card: Boo-hiss)* and his icky-sticky dudes were pretty quiet. Nobody could see them because they were very good at hiding. Why, they were so good at hiding, they were invisible! They waited for just the right time to attack. Was Cowboy Healthy Smile *(Flash card: Wow!)* doomed to be captured by Boss Plaque *(Flash card: Boo-hiss)* forever? Yikes!

Cowboy Healthy Smile *(Flash card: Wow!)* could sense that something dangerous was about to happen. He yelled for help! To his rescue came our hero, Sheriff Smilin' Sam *(Flash card: To the rescue!)* with his strong but gentle brush, Buster. Sheriff Smilin' Sam *(Flash card: To the rescue!)* used Buster to give Boss Plaque *(Flash card: Boo-hiss)* and his icky-sticky dudes the old brush-off. Buster was very good at busting up the plaque gang! But Boss Plaque *(Flash card: Boo-hiss)* and the icky-sticky dudes were pretty tough. They knew how to hide from Buster!

They were tough, but not too tough for Sheriff Smilin' Sam *(Flash card: To the rescue!)*. No siree! He attacked the icky-sticky villains with a clever rope trick called Flossing. With his flossing know-how, Sheriff Smilin' Sam *(Flash card: To the rescue!)* could round up those sneaky hiding critters and move them out!

Now Sheriff Smilin' Sam *(Flash card: To the rescue!)* didn't leave Cowboy Healthy Smile *(Flash card: Wow!)* without extra protection. No siree! Deputy Fluoride *(Flash card: Hurray!)* saved the day. Cowboy Healthy Smile *(Flash card: Wow!)* and the town of Open Wide were saved from another attack by Boss Plaque *(Flash card: Boo-hiss!)* and his icky-sticky dudes!

Follow-up Activities: Trouble in Open Wide

After reading the melodrama, ask students to:

- List the three functions of teeth.
- Describe the role of plaque in the decay process.
- Name three things we can do to help prevent decay. *(Brush, floss, use fluoride.)*
- State the effect of fluoride on the teeth.
- Ask the students whether Boss Plaque comes back another time.
- Have the students try to find their way through the Deputy Fluoride maze (see handout).

TOOTH-TAC-TOE GAME

This game uses the typical review questions present earlier in this lesson to test students' knowledge of the dental information presented during the year.

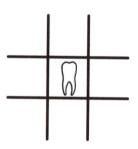

Directions

1. Draw a tic-tac-toe game square on the black/white board.
2. Divide the class into two teams, Molars and Incisors.
3. Ask the first player on the Molar team a question from the review list of typical questions presented earlier in this lesson. If the player answers correctly, the team can draw a molar in a square of their choice. If the answer is incorrect, no mark can be made.
4. Now it is the Incisors' turn. Ask the first player on the Incisors team a question from the dental review. Follow the procedure in step 3, but have the team draw an incisor in the square of their choice.
5. Continue the game until one team has a series of molars or incisors in a horizontal, vertical, or diagonal line on the board.
6. The teams can replay with different questions to finish the review of the lesson.

Suggestions

- Have the two teams use different colored chalk or erasable marker on the board, as the molars and incisors may look alike.
- For grades 4–6, substitute more difficult questions.

STOP THE PIRATES GAME

This game uses the typical review questions presented earlier in this lesson to test students' knowledge of the dental information presented during the year.

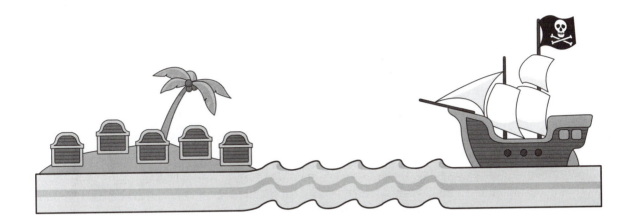

Directions

1. On the black/white board, draw five treasure chests on an island and a pirate ship off shore. Between the island and the pirate ship are five waves of water. The water is keeping the pirates from reaching the island and the treasure.
2. Divide the class into two teams, Pirates and Guards. The Pirates want to take the treasure and the Guards want to hide it.
3. Ask the first player on the Pirates team a question from the review list of typical questions presented earlier in this lesson. If the answer is correct, the Pirates can remove (erase) one wave. If the answer is incorrect, no waves can be removed.
4. Next, ask a question of the first player on the Guards team. If the player answers correctly, one treasure chest can be buried (erased). If the answer is incorrect, no chests can be buried.
5. The game continues until the Pirates remove the five waves of water or the Guards bury the five treasure chests.

Suggestions

- Use colored chalk or erasable markers to draw the picture on the board.
- For grades 4–6, add more waves and more treasure chests, and substitute more difficult questions.

PICTURE QUIZ

Using the handout of the train picture at the end of this lesson, have students find the five items in the picture that will keep their teeth healthy.

DENTAL IQ QUIZ

Using the quiz handout at the end of this lesson, test students' knowledge of the dental information presented during the year.

TOOTH SLEUTH GAME

Have students use the tooth sleuth handout at the end of this lesson to discover individuals in the classroom who follow good dental practices.

BLACKBOARD FOOTBALL GAME

This game uses the typical review questions presented earlier in this lesson to test students' knowledge of the dental information presented during the year.

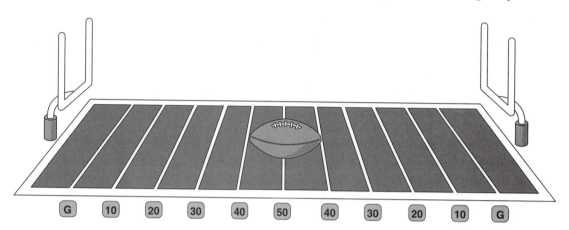

Directions

1. Draw a football field on the black/white board. Mark a goal post at either end and indicate the various yard lines (10, 20, 30, 40, 50, 40, 30, 20, 10). Draw a football on the 50-yard line.
2. Divide the class into two teams (e.g., the Haunted Mouths and the Buzzard Breaths).
3. Ask one of the Haunted Mouth players a question from the review list of typical questions presented earlier in this lesson. If the player answers correctly, the football is moved (drawn) so that it is on the Buzzard Breaths' 40-yard line.
4. Next, ask a Buzzard Breath player a question. If the player answers correctly, the ball is pushed back 10 yards to the 50-yard line again.
5. If a player gives an incorrect answer, the ball does not move.
6. The first team that reaches the opponent's goal line has made a touchdown and receives 6 points.
7. A scorekeeper can score the game as shown:

HAUNTED MOUTH	BUZZARD BREATH
6	6
6	0
12	6

8. The game ends when all of the review questions have been asked.

Suggestions

Use colored chalk or erasable markers to draw the football field, football, and field goals on the board.

Closure

(2–3 minutes)

- Restate the objectives in question form.
- Check students' knowledge and understanding of the concepts presented.
- If time permits, address any other questions the students may have.

LeSSon plaN / LAST VISIT

GRADE LEVEL _____ ROOM _____

SCHOOL _____ TEACHER _____

TIME REQUIRED (30 MINUTES) _____

Preparation in Classroom _____

_____

_____

_____

_____

Anticipatory Planning _____

_____

_____

_____

_____

_____

_____

_____

Review of Previous Objectives: _____

_____

_____

_____

_____

_____

Three Specific Objectives:

1. _____

_____

2. _____

_____

3. _____

LeJJoN pLqN / **LAST VISIT** *continues*

Information to Be Presented Will Include:

(Topics) _____

_____

_____

_____

_____

_____

(Methods) _____

_____

_____

_____

_____

_____

(Lecture, demonstration, visual aids, group discussion) _____

_____

_____

_____

_____

_____

Guided Practice Activities _____

_____

_____

_____

_____

_____

Closure _____

_____

_____

_____

_____

_____

_____

Try to find your way through the Deputy Fluoride maze.

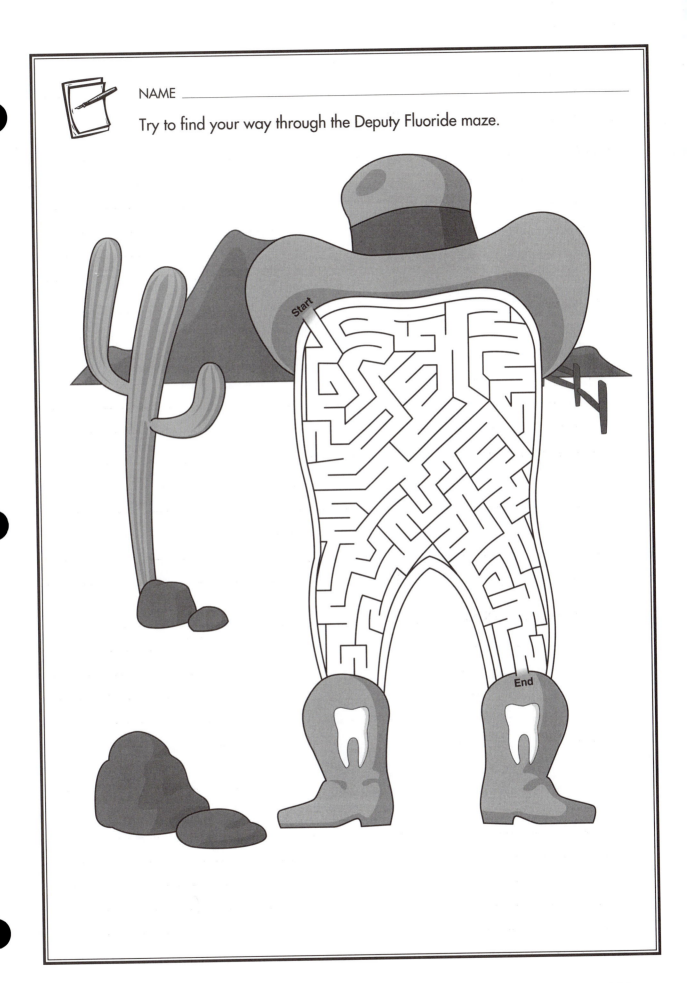

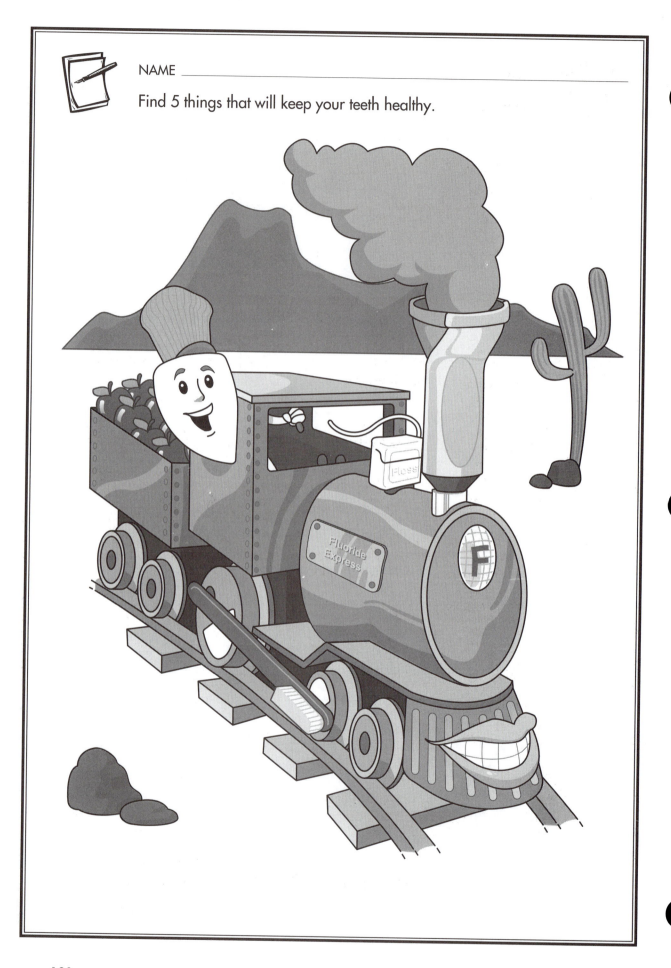

NAME _____

Find 5 things that will keep your teeth healthy.

NAME _____

Dental IQ Quiz

Circle the correct answer (true or false) for the following questions.

1. You don't always need to take good care of baby teeth since they will fall out anyway.

   True   False

2. Flossing your teeth is just as important as brushing them.

   True   False

3. It's important to eat a variety of good foods every day.

   True   False

4. You should brush your tongue daily.

   True   False

Circle the best answer for the following questions.

5. The best way to brush your teeth is:

   Up and down   Scrub hard   Wiggle jiggle

6. Which is a sign of gingivitis?

   Tooth decay   Missing teeth   Bleeding gums

7. A sticky film of bacteria that forms on your teeth is called:

   Plaque   Tartar   Gingivitis

8. Fluoride can be found in:

   Toothpaste   Toothbrushes   Crackers

NAME _____

Find someone who. . . . . .

Quietly ask your classmates and teacher if they fit the description in any of the boxes below. If they do, ask them to put their name in the square.

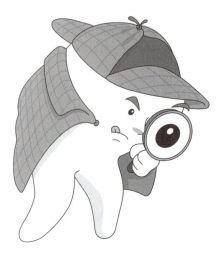

Tooth Sleuth

Find someone who has a cavity.	Find someone who has braces.	Find someone who has floss in his or her desk.
Find someone who has fresh fruit in his or her lunch. (What kind?)	Find someone who eats a cereal that doesn't have any sugar added to it. (What kind?)	Find someone who brushes three times a day.
Find someone who has been to see the dentist in the past month.	Find someone who is missing a tooth.	Find someone who uses a fluoride rinse at home. (What kind?)

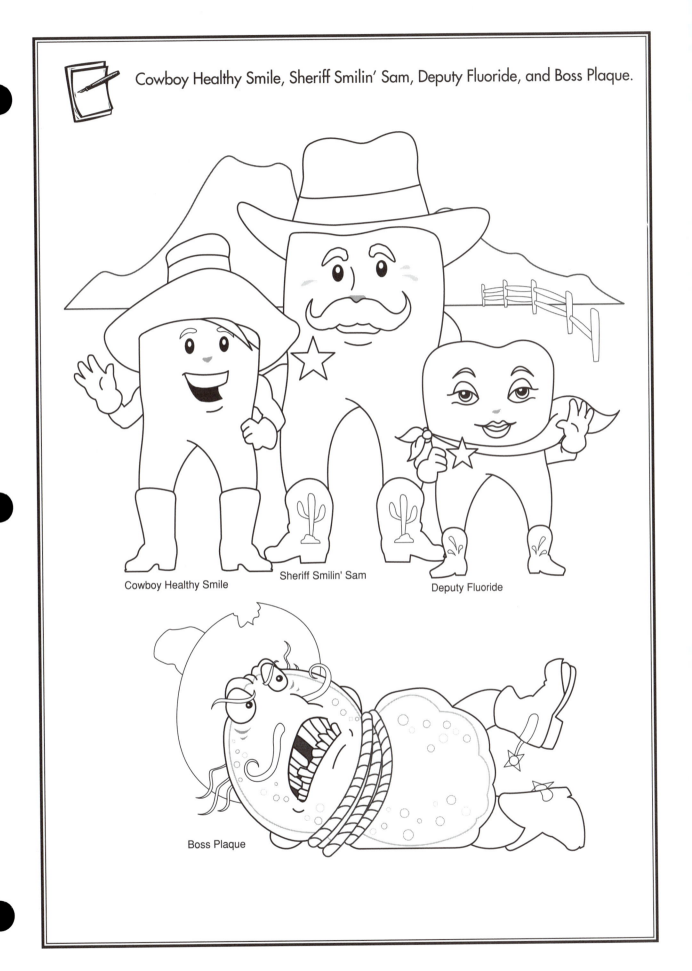

Cowboy Healthy Smile, Sheriff Smilin' Sam, Deputy Fluoride, and Boss Plaque.

Cowboy Healthy Smile

Sheriff Smilin' Sam

Deputy Fluoride

Boss Plaque

Children With Special Needs*

For legal purposes, pupils with special education needs should be designated "individuals with special needs." This designation should include only those pupils whose educational needs cannot be met by the regular classroom teacher with modifications of the regular school program, and who will benefit from special instruction and/or services. This chapter can serve as a reference when incorporating preventive education lesson plans into a classroom in which some or all individuals have special needs. The lesson plans presented earlier in Section Two should be adapted and modified as needed to meet the needs of these learners.

The purpose of special education is to develop educational programs to help children with special needs to achieve the greatest possible self-sufficiency and success in the classroom. Dental health educators may encounter these children in the following settings:

- Closed-campus programs: The school's student population is made up of only special needs children ranging in age from 3 to 21 years and with various handicapping conditions. Most closed-campus programs specifically address the physically challenged child.
- Self-contained classroom programs/special day classes: The classroom is located on the regular school campus and may provide some mainstreaming opportunities for special needs students.
- Mainstreamed programs: Special needs children are integrated into the regular classrooms for the entire day. Modifications may be necessary or additional attention may be needed.

Several categories of special needs/special education classes may be provided in these programs, among them: autistic, developmentally delayed, hearing impaired, independent living skills, learning handicapped, physically handicapped, severely emotionally disturbed, and speech impaired. The following subclassifications may also be specified: communicatively handicapped, cerebral palsy, and severely handicapped.

The following suggestions are provided to help the dental health educator meet the needs of the special needs students in the classroom.

- Teach learning tasks in small steps, and sequence them in the proper order, one skill at a time.
- Check for knowledge at each step. Use repetition.
- If applicable, have students repeat orally what they have learned.
- Use different motivational strategies.
- Use a consistent and familiar structure when presenting information.
- Provide consistent reinforcement, especially in the development of new skills.
- Assess progress on a regular basis by checking for understanding and ability to perform the skills taught.
- Use visuals from the classroom such as puppets, toothbrushes, tooth models, etc., where possible.

*Courtesy of Kate Varanelli, RDH, MS, Sacramento SBIII

- Provide continuous and immediate feedback for all activities.
- Invite caregivers, where applicable, to participate.

Dental neglect among students with special needs is often very high. The importance of dental care should be emphasized to caretakers, parents, and teachers. The remainder of this lesson presents information that can be used to improve the dental health of students with special needs. Use these suggestions when implementing the guided practice activities of brushing, flossing, and using fluoride in the classroom. Special positioning options are also presented.

Brushing

For the child with special needs, suggest that the teacher use the process of brushing to help meet other needs such as:

- Improving fine motor skills
- Teaching the parts of the mouth and their functions
- Improving language development
- Teaching self-help skills
- Teaching colors (toothbrushes comes in many different colors [red, blue, green, orange, yellow])

The type of toothbrush and toothbrushing method should be geared to each individual's needs and ability (some have gripper or rubber ends to help with dexterity). Some students may not like having a foreign object, such as a toothbrush, placed in their mouths. You may have to work on desensitizing the child before thorough brushing can be accomplished.

Use a small toothbrush. Repetition and sequencing are very important. Emphasize the need to always start in one area of the mouth and end in a certain area to ensure that all areas have been brushed, and to instill the habit of thorough brushing right from the start.

When teaching step-by-step brushing, emphasize the steps in Figure 2–13.

If the child gags easily or can't expectorate, brush with a fluoride rinse instead of toothpaste. First, brush without the rinse. Then, pour a little rinse into a cup, dip the toothbrush into it, and brush with the rinse.

If total or partial assistance is needed, try to empower the child in some other way. Modifications or attachments may be necessary to adapt a toothbrush for a child with a physical impairment (see Fig. 2–14).

Flossing

Only those students with the necessary coordination should participate in flossing. However, the importance of flossing should be covered. Emphasize that brushing is not enough. Flossing is needed to remove plaque between the teeth, where a toothbrush can't reach. Daily rinsing with a fluoride rinse can give the child additional protection against cavities by strengthening tooth enamel.

When teaching flossing, emphasize the steps in Figure 2–15.

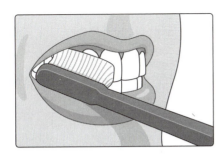

Place toothbrush bristles at the gum line, at a 45-degree angle to the teeth and gums. Press gently using short vibrating strokes, back-and-forth, or light "wiggle jiggle" motion. Start in the upper right quadrant at the last tooth, brushing the outside.

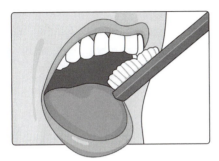

Move all the way around to the last tooth on the opposite side; then move to the inside and finish with the chewing surfaces. Do the same for the lower teeth. Be sure to brush each tooth.

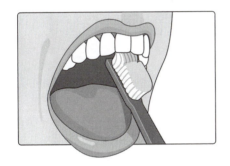

To clean the inside surfaces of the front teeth, both upper and lower, hold the brush vertically with the end of the toothbrush and bristles vertically at a 45-degree angle to the toothbrush and gums.

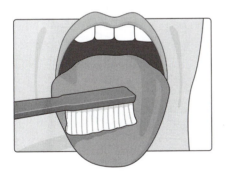

Don't forget to brush the top of your tongue, too, as it can harbor many bacteria. Move the toothbrush bristles with flat long strokes from the back of your tongue to the front end (stick your tongue out for this step).

FIGURE 2–13 Step-by-step brushing.

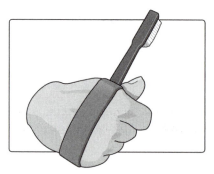

Attach the brush to the child's hand with a wide elastic band.

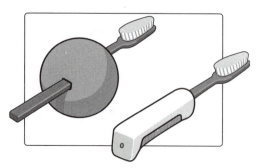

For children with a limited grasp, enlarge the brush handle with a sponge, rubber ball, or bicycle handle grip.

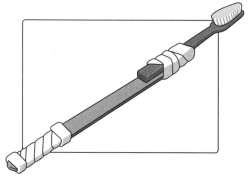

For children who can't raise their hand or arm, lengthen the brush handle with a ruler, tongue depressor, or long wooden spoon.

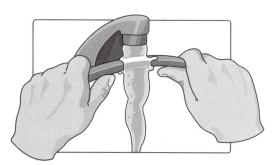

Bend the brush handle by running hot water over the handle (not the head) of the brush.

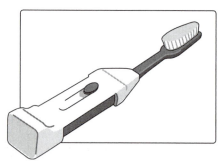

For children who can't manipulate a regular toothbrush, providing an electric toothbrush may enable them to brush by themselves.

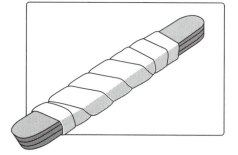

If the child can't keep his or her mouth open, use a mouth prop—for example, three or four tongue depressors taped together, a rolled-up moistened washcloth, or a rubber doorstop. (Emphasize that teachers and parents should always ask a dental professional how to use a mouth prop to avoid injuring a child's mouth.)

FIGURE 2–14 Methods for adapting a toothbrush. (*Adapted from an original publication by Johnson and Johnson.*)

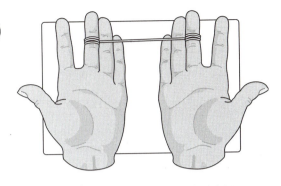

Take an 18-inch piece of floss and wind it around the middle finger of each hand. Or, tie the ends together in a circle.

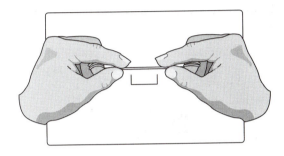

Grasp the floss firmly between the thumb and index finger of each hand. Hold a half-inch section taut for more control. Work it gently between the teeth until it reaches the gum line.

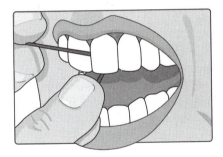

Curve the floss into a C-shape around a tooth. Slide the floss gently up and down the side of the tooth. Remove the floss gently and repeat for all teeth. Take care not to injure the gums with the floss.

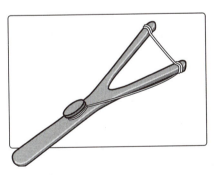

Flossing requires some degree of coordination and takes practice. It may help to use a floss holder.

FIGURE 2–15 Step-by-step flossing.

Fluoride

Depending on the fluoride level in the area's water supply, the appropriate method of fluoride supplementation should be used. If the child will not tolerate a fluoride rinse or tablet, an alternative method should be tried. It may take a while before a child accepts the fluoride.

When teaching the use of a fluoride rinse, emphasize the steps in Fig. 2–16.

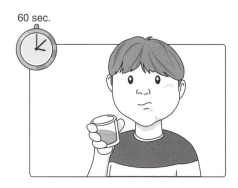

Have the child take the recommended dose of a fluoride rinse (usually a capful), swish it around in the mouth for 60 seconds, and then rinse out, taking care not to swallow it. To get full fluoride protection, the child shouldn't eat or drink for 30 minutes after rinsing.

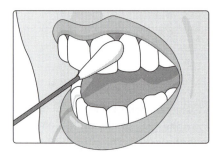

If the child is unable to rinse without swallowing, use a cotton swab or a toothbrush to place a little fluoride rinse on the child's teeth. The child's dental professional may also recommend a prescription fluoride gel treatment.

FIGURE 2–16 Step-by-step rinsing.

Positioning

If a caretaker is responsible for brushing the student's teeth, review the use of alternative positions, which can make the procedure comfortable for both the child and the caretaker. Emphasize the importance of choosing a position that supports the child's head, allows the caretaker to see well, and ensures ease of manipulation during the procedure. If in doubt, the caretaker should always ask a dental professional which is the safest, most comfortable position for the child. Emphasize the need to use care to prevent the child from choking or gagging when the head is tilted back (see Figure 2–17).

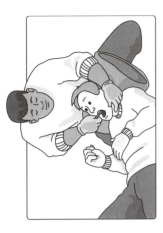

Lying on the Floor
Have the child lie on the floor with his or her head on a pillow. You should kneel behind the child's head. You can use your arm to hold the child still.

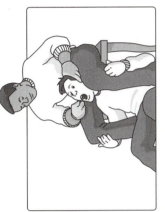

Sitting on the Floor
Have the child sit on the floor; you should sit behind the child on a chair. Have the child lean his or her head against your knees. If the child is uncooperative or uncontrollable, you can place your legs over the child's arms to keep the child still.

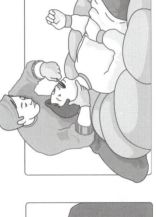

In a Beanbag Chair
For children who have difficulty sitting up straight, a beanbag chair lets them relax without fear of falling. Use the same position as for a bed or sofa.

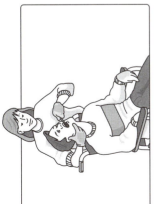

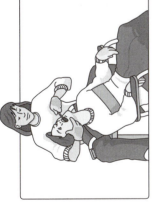

For the Child in a Wheelchair
Stand behind the wheelchair. Use your arm to brace the child's head against the chair or your body. Use a pillow for the child's comfort. Or, sit behind the wheelchair. Remember to lock the chair wheels first, then tilt the chair back into your lap.

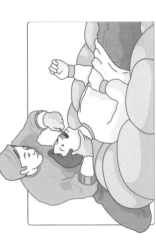

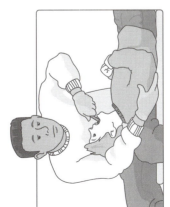

On a Bed or Sofa
Have the child lie on a bed or sofa with his or her head in your lap. Support the child's head and shoulders with your arm. If the child is uncooperative or uncontrollable, a second person can hold the child's hands or feet, if needed.

FIGURE 2–17 Alternate positions for providing dental care.

Le**ss**on pl**a**n / CHILD WITH SPECIAL NEEDS

GRADE LEVEL Special Education _____ ROOM _____

SCHOOL _____ TEACHER _____

TIME REQUIRED (30 MINUTES) _____

Preparation in Classroom _____

_____

_____

_____

_____

_____

Anticipatory Planning _____

_____

_____

_____

_____

_____

_____

_____

Review of Previous Objectives: _____

_____

_____

_____

_____

_____

Three Specific Objectives:

1. _____

_____

2. _____

_____

3. _____

_____

Information to Be Presented Will Include:

(Topics) _____

_____

_____

_____

_____

_____

(Methods) _____

_____

_____

_____

_____

_____

(Lecture, demonstration, visual aids, group discussion) _____

_____

_____

_____

_____

_____

Guided Practice Activities _____

_____

_____

_____

_____

_____

Closure _____

_____

_____

_____

_____

_____

_____

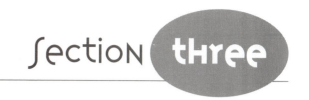

ſection **three**

Creating a Community Outreach Program

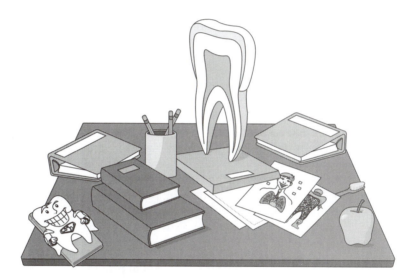

this section outlines an approach to preparing for a community outreach program and provides two sample programs. Dental health professionals can play an important role by participating in community outreach programs. Your participation will give the community an opportunity to explore various topics, careers, and issues surrounding dental health and education. Before volunteering or committing to participate in a community outreach program, you will need to get organized, target resources, secure educational materials, and implement and evaluate the program.

The following outline can provide a guideline to assist you as you prepare for your community outreach program.

Organization

To begin, you need to set an objective or goal for the program. Your planning should include the following components:

- Date and time
- Location (indoors or outdoors)
- Size of the group participating
- Equipment required (e.g., tables, chairs, blackboard, easel, audiovisual)
- Staff or volunteers needed (proportionate to group size, recruitment)

- In-service training requirements (preplanning, training to outline responsibilities, goals)
- Advertisement or publicity needed or provided if held in conjuction with another event (see handout at end of this section)

Resources

Identify various organizations and groups that you can contact for supplies and information. These might include:

- National, state, and local dental hygienists associations
- National, state, and local dental associations
- National, state, and local dental assisting associations
- Dental hygiene, dental, and dental assisting schools
- Community service groups
- Dental supply companies (Smart Practice, Henry Schein, etc.)
- Local and county public health services
- Oral Health Professional Sales distributors (Colgate, Procter & Gamble, Oral B, Johnson and Johnson, etc.)

Educational Materials

All materials developed for your program should:

- Be age-appropriate
- Be multilingual, if appropriate for the community (e.g., in English and Spanish)
- Use universal signage (simple, clear symbols and drawings)
- Make use of visual aids (e.g., posters, models, toothbrushes, floss)
- Avoid copyright infringement

Implementation

To carry out the program, you will need to provide for the following components:

- An outline of the program time schedule
- Advertisement/Publicity
- Delegation of duties (stations, monitors, coordinators, etc.) during the program
- A list of supplies and other materials needed for the presentation
- Transportation and storage of supplies
- Set up
- Break down

Evaluation

After you have presented the program, you will want to evaluate the outcome to determine the success of your efforts.

- Whether you met your goals
- How well participants have learned and retained the information presented
- Whether a behavior change was exhibited
- Whether a decrease in decay can be noted from previous examinations

The remainder of this section consists of specific guidelines for presenting two types of outreach programs: a dental health fair and a parent education meeting. Remember, the most successful outcomes are always a result of advance planning.

Community Outreach Program: Dental Health Fair

Courtesy of U.O.P. Janet Chan Fricke

Preparation

(1-hour in-service training)

Recruit volunteers from the dental professions to assist in the health fair (students in dental programs as well as members in the professional dental organizations within the community). Provide in-service training for the volunteers to familiarize them with the program and with their responsibilities. If workable, assign each new volunteer to a team in which one member has previous outreach experience and acts as a mentor to the rest of the team. Working in teams makes it easier to carry out activities at each station, especially with nonprofessional volunteers.

Children and parents visiting the dental health fair will walk through each station. Obtain samples of toothbrushes, floss, stickers, and other supplies several months in advance; these can then be given away to participants during the fair.

Anticipatory Planning

(15 minutes)

- Review the instructions.
- Introduce presenters.
- Describe the goals of the program or the format of information to be covered at each station. If space or number of volunteers is limited, you can combine the stations to fit your needs.
- Review break and lunch times.
- Review the locations of emergency and restroom facilities.
- Have a resource and referral list available at Station 6 for parents.

Instruction/Information

(5–10 minutes per station)

In the following sample program, six stations are set up to discuss various topics relating to dental health. A dental screening is held at the last station, with a prize (sticker) given to children who complete the screening. Depending on the needs of your community, you may wish to or substitute other topics.

Station   Topic
1. Visiting the dentist; dental tools
2. Diet and nutrition
3. Decay process and fluoride
4. Toothbrushing and flossing
5. Oral injury prevention and the dental emergency
6. Dental screening and prize

More than one topic may be included at each station.

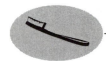

(5–10 minutes per station)

Guided Practice Activities

STATION 1: VISITING THE DENTIST; DENTAL TOOLS

Volunteers should explain what children will encounter on their first visit to the dentist. Among the areas to be covered at this station are:

- Introduction of the dentist, dental hygienist, and dental assistant
- What happens at the first visit
- The dental chart (a book about each child)
- Use of gloves, mask, eye protection, and gowns for infection control
- Radiographic pictures of the teeth and bone, panorex, bitewings, periapicial, etc.

Volunteers can demonstrate typical instruments and explain terminology (refer to the glossary and the tooth talk terminology listing in the appendix for definitions of dental terminology). Among the items to be exhibited are:

- Patient hand mirror
- Mouth mirror
- Tooth counter (explorer)
- Straw or Mr. Slurpy (saliva ejector)
- Electric toothbrush (slow speed with disposable prophy angle)
- Large tooth model
- Tooth model with restorations (silver star, silver hat, sealants)

Visuals: A variety of infection control items used in the dental office; a tray of dental instruments (see preceding listing); and models.

STATION 2: DIET AND NUTRITION

Volunteers should be able to help children identify healthy foods and compare them to foods that are not healthy. Among the areas to be covered at this station are:

- The food pyramid and recommended servings
- Healthy foods (a basket of different foods can be provided; the children can then be asked to identify the healthy foods)

Visuals: Charts, posters, and handouts of the food pyramid and nutrition or diet-related facts. Consult your local dairy counsel for additional information.

STATION 3: THE DECAY PROCESS AND FLUORIDE

Volunteers should be able to teach about the decay process and describe how a cavity starts. They should explain how fluoride can strengthen teeth, making them more resistant to decay.

Decay Process
- Explain the decay process:
  Plaque + Sugar = Acid
  Acid + Healthy tooth = Decay (cavities)
- Describe baby bottle tooth decay. Explain how the decay process is accelerated when milk, formula, juice, or breast milk in a bottle is allowed to remain in a baby's mouth. Explain when and how to wean infants off the bottle. Recommend dilution of juices and use of water in bottles.

- Using a large molar model, show how a small pit and fissure cavity can quickly enlarge into a big cavity that may cause discomfort.
- Using a model of two teeth, show how interproximal decay occurs.
- Show how disclosing tablets and solution can detect plaque on teeth.

Fluoride

- Describe how fluoride (a "tooth vitamin") can prevent tooth decay by making the tooth more resistant (strengthening the enamel). Explain that fluoride can be found in some foods and water. It may also be applied to teeth at the dentist's office.
- Highlight the different ways to receive fluoride: water, toothpaste, mouth rinse, tablets, and fluoride treatments at the dentist's office.

Visuals: Pictures of the decay process, decayed teeth, and baby bottle tooth decay; disclosing tablets and solution; patient mirrors; and various products containing fluoride. Pictures and videotapes may be available through the local dental society.

STATION 4: TOOTHBRUSHING AND FLOSSING

Volunteers should demonstrate how to choose a soft bristle toothbrush and the proper brushing technique. They should show examples of different types of floss and demonstrate proper flossing technique on a tooth model or in their mouth.

Toothbrushing

- Describe and provide examples of different types of toothbrushes (hard versus soft, small versus large, single and multi-side).
- Emphasize the need for one toothbrush per person (don't share).
- Describe the qualities of a good toothbrush versus one that is worn out.
- Demonstrate the proper technique: brushing at a 45-degree angle to the gum line; using small, circular strokes angled into the gum line for the front and back of teeth; and using circular strokes on the chewing surfaces.
- Emphasize the need to brush the tongue after the teeth to remove bacteria on the tongue.

Flossing

- Demonstrate proper flossing technique, including the appropriate length of floss and finger positioning.
- Emphasize the need for adult supervision.
- Demonstrate use of a floss holder.
- Discuss and provide examples of types of floss available (children's flavor, mint fluoride, tape, waxed, unwaxed, and superfloss)

Visuals: A large tooth model, large toothbrush, pictures of proper toothbrushing and flossing technique, a variety of toothbrushes and floss. Hand out samples, if available, to participants.

STATION 5: ORAL INJURY PREVENTION AND THE DENTAL EMERGENCY

Volunteers should stress the importance of preventing oral injury by wearing a mouth guard for all contact sports and activities in which there is a risk of oral injury (baseball, basketball, football, soccer, in-line skating, skateboards, hockey, wrestling, etc.). They should also describe the types of mouth guards available and provide examples:

- Boil and bite: Purchased in a sporting goods store; softened in boiling water, then bitten down on to form an impression of the teeth; available in limited sizes and provides only limited coverage to the tops of teeth
- Custom-fit: Made directly from a mold of the athlete's teeth; fits better, lasts longer (less distortion)

Dental Emergency Procedures

Volunteers should be able to describe the first aid that should be provided for the following common dental emergencies. Refer to the lesson on Dental Safety and Oral Injury Prevention in Section Two for specific instructions to be given for each emergency.

- Bitten tongue
- Broken tooth
- Knocked-out tooth
- Objects wedged between the teeth
- Orthodontia problems
- Possible fractured jaw
- Toothache

Visuals: A variety of mouth guards and a large chart or poster describing dental emergency procedures. Handouts may be available through the local dental society.

STATION 6: DENTAL SCREENING AND PRIZE

A "look-and-see" screening for obvious dental problems will be done, and parents will be informed of any problems or needs identified. Complete screenings are not done during this session, and this visit does not take the place of a dental examination. Volunteers should be able to identify common dental problems and help reinforce good dental habits. Among the areas to be addressed at this station are:

- Ways to keep teeth happy and healthy, including regular visits to the dentist, healthy food choices, and good oral hygiene habits (brushing and flossing)
- Referral to the child's dentist if he or she needs immediate dental care or give a referral list. (Orthodontics and routine dental care are not considered emergencies necessitating immediate care.)

Give a sticker (prize) to each child who participates so you know who has completed the "look-and-see" screening.

Closure

(2–3 minutes at each station)

- Check participants' knowledge and understanding of the concepts presented.
- If time permits, address any other questions participants may have.

cHecklist / DENTAL HEALTH FAIR

_____ Provide in-service training

_____ Obtain supplies

_____ Assign specific stations and shifts

_____ Reserve equipment (tables, VCR, monitor, videotapes, etc.)

_____ Notify volunteers:

      _____ What to bring

      _____ What to wear

      _____ What time

      _____ Location

      _____ Coordinator's phone number(s)

      _____ Other

Comments: _____

Community Outreach Program: Parent Education Meeting

Preparation

(5 minutes before beginning lesson) Display a variety of pacifiers; pictures of baby bottle tooth decay; infant-sized and other toothbrushes; fluoride drops, tablets, and rinses; floss; models; flip-charts; and a chart or handout of the food pyramid.

Anticipatory Planning

(5 minutes)
- Review the previous presentation, if applicable.
- Introduce presenters.
- Describe the goal of the presentation: To educate parents about early child-hood oral health care, prevention, and feeding practices.

General Objectives

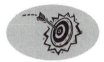

State specifically no more than three or four objectives appropriate for the audi-ence that indicate what the majority of the attendees will be able to achieve by the completion of the program. Examples include:

(2–3 minutes)
- Describe the dental decay process.
- Identify the causes of baby bottle tooth decay and how to prevent it.
- Recognize early infant oral habits and know how to modify or correct them.
- Utilize new information to make wise oral health decisions for their chil-dren.

Instruction/Information

(40–60 minutes) More than one topic may be included or combined with the guided practice seg-ment (30 minutes).

- Discuss dental problems of early infancy, and dental disease among the school-age population.
- Present information on preventing baby bottle tooth decay.
- Describe the causes of tooth decay and how it can be prevented.
- Discuss bedtime routines, use of pacifiers, and thumbsucking.
- Equate dental care with future smiles; discuss when to see a dentist, and how to find one.

Dental problems of early infancy

Cavities and gum disease are the most common health problems seen in children. Cavities and gum disease are serious problems. Gum disease causes the gums to become red, sore, and puffy, and bleed easily. Cavities and gum disease can cause pain and infection. Cavities in the baby teeth are just as serious as cavities in the permanent teeth. If baby teeth are lost too early, children don't learn to speak correctly, have difficulties with chewing, and the permanent teeth can come in crooked.

Ask parents, "Have any of you heard of baby bottle tooth decay?" Explain that it is a condition that occurs when a baby is put to bed with a bottle or allowed to walk around with a bottle in the mouth that contains any liquid other than water. The pooling of sugary liquid in the baby's mouth causes severe cavities when left for long periods of time. The teeth can even rot down to the gums *(show visual)*. This is a serious and painful problem. The best way to prevent this from happening is to hold a baby while feeding and to avoid putting the baby to bed with a bottle. Explain that you will be teaching other ways to prevent baby bottle tooth decay, such as toothbrushing, during this presentation.

Causes of decay

Discuss what causes decay and how it can be prevented. Include the following topics:

- The decay process (see Fig. 2–1)
- Cleaning, brushing, and flossing needs of children from early infancy through the teenage years (have samples of toothbrushes available to hand out to parents)
- Benefits of fluoride
- Nutrition for dental health

Dental Disease Process

Explain that cavities and gum disease are both caused by germs growing on the teeth. When these germs group together, they are called plaque *(show visual)*.

Proper Brushing

Describe the importance of brushing as a way to break up plaque germs and prevent gum disease and cavities, even baby bottle tooth decay. Review proper brushing technique.

Pick a toothbrush with a soft bristle and a small head *(show examples appropriate for a child, teenager, and adult)*. Demonstrate brushing on a Typodont (large tooth model), using small, circular strokes, and establishing a pattern. Pass out toothbrushes to those who would like them. Tell parents that before a baby has teeth, they should use a soft, clean cloth to clean the baby's gums. Explain that parents of toddlers should brush their teeth at least once a day to begin to develop the habit of brushing. Caution that children aged 2 years and under should not use toothpaste when brushing because they swallow it.

Finally, tell parents, "You can help your child have healthier teeth by encouraging him or her to brush before school, after snacks, and before bed."

From bottle to cup: Preventing baby bottle tooth decay

Prolonged bottle feeding can lead to tooth decay. It can also promote overfeeding and prevent the baby from getting other needed nutrients from the diet.

By 7 to 9 months of age, a baby may be ready to learn to drink from a cup. At this age, a baby is developmentally able to sit up with support, grasp and hold objects, and coordination is improving. This is the ideal time to introduce the cup. Some babies are suddenly ready to give up the bottle or show an interest in learning. If this happens, parents should take advantage of the opportunity.

Parents should begin by replacing one bottle feeding a day with a cup feeding. The meal at which the baby is most alert and rested is best or whenever he or she begins to show most interest. Tell parents not to expect the baby to know what to do at first. Parents should help by lifting the cup to the baby's mouth, tipping it to give the baby a small drink. In time, the baby will learn to do this by himself or herself. After a few days or weeks, parents can replace a second bottle feeding with a cup feeding at a second meal or at snacktime. They should continue to replace bottle feedings until the baby is no longer drinking from a bottle.

The baby may be fussy until he or she gets used to this new experience. Parents should be prepared for dribbling and spills. It may be messy at first, but emphasize that parents should take things slowly and be patient. Always reward the baby's success with kisses and cheerful words.

Emphasize that when choosing a cup, parents should choose one that is small and easy for the baby to lift and hold. The cup should be unbreakable. Some "training cups" have handles and a lid with a spout; others have a weighted bottom or a wide base to help prevent messy spills. Caution parents not to fill the cup to the top; they should pour only until it is half full.

Readiness to drink from a cup doesn't mean that the baby is ready to drink cow's milk. Parents should continue to use formula. Cow's milk should not be offered until the child's physician or other health care provider recommends it.

Finally, emphasize that it is best to introduce juices in a cup, not the bottle. Diluted juices can first be introduced at about 7 months of age. By 12 to 18 months, the baby should be drinking from a cup instead of a bottle. If parents have concerns related to weaning, they should discuss them with their pediatrician or other health care provider.

Bedtime routines

Emphasize the importance of starting good oral health habits at an early age. Parents should establish a routine of brushing teeth before bed by the time a child reaches 1½ years of age. Discuss issues related to use of pacifiers and thumbsucking.

Pacifiers

Discuss the variety of pacifiers available (orthodontic, etc.) and instructions for their use. Caution parents never to tie a pacifier around a baby's neck. Present the following guidelines for choosing a pacifier:*

- Look for a sturdy, one-piece construction, and a flexible, nontoxic material.
- Be sure the pacifier is too large to be swallowed.
- Make sure the shield or mouth guard portion cannot be separated from the nipple.
- Look for two ventilating holes.

Thumb Sucking Habits

Advise parents that children should stop sucking their thumbs by the age of 2 to 3 years. The earlier it is stopped, the better, and the less damage it will do. Preferably thumb sucking will stop before the permanent teeth erupt (lower incisors). Caution parents that the longer the child maintains the habit, the greater the risk of improperly positioned teeth.

Discussion: Future smiles

Discuss when to see a dentist and how to find one. Have available resources for care in the local area. Advise parents that the child's first appointment for a healthy dental checkup should occur between 6 months and 1 year of age to review fluoride content, vitamin supplements, baby bottle or breast feeding practice, etc.

*Guidelines for safe use of pacifiers by Dr. Arthur J. Nowak.

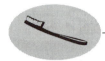

(30 minutes)

Guided Practice Activities

This segment may be combined with the preceding instruction/information segment. Visual aids are included at the end of the lesson.

Areas that might be presented in an activity format include proper toothbrushing and flossing technique, use of fluoride and sealants, and proper nutrition. This segment might utilize small group discussion or a question-and-answer session. Provide handouts for the dental health topics covered (see end of lesson and appendix).

TOPICS FOR PARENT TEACHING

Reinforce the following information for parents, using visual aids and demonstrating proper techniques. Provide written dental health information that parents can take with them and refer to later (see handouts at the end of this lesson).

Toothbrushing

Describe and provide examples of different types of toothbrushes (hard versus soft, small versus large, single and multi-side). Emphasize the need for one toothbrush per person (don't share). Describe the qualities of a good toothbrush versus one that is worn out. Demonstrate the proper technique: brushing at a 45-degree angle to the gum line; using small, circular strokes angled into the gum line for the front and back of teeth; and using circular strokes on the chewing surfaces. Emphasize the need to brush the tongue after the teeth to remove bacteria on the tongue.

Flossing

Show various samples of floss. Explain that parents need to floss children's teeth to remove the plaque that builds up between the teeth where the toothbrush cannot reach. Younger children should floss with parent guidance at least once a day. Floss holders may also be used. Demonstrate proper flossing, and have samples available for audience participation.

Fluoride

Explain that fluoride makes teeth stronger and helps prevent cavities. Hold up a glass of water as you explain that although certain foods contain fluoride (e.g., fish, green leafy vegetables, apples), the most cost-effective way to get fluoride is in water. When a community's water undergoes fluoridation, the right amount of fluoride is added to the water to prevent cavities. If the water is not fluoridated, parents should ask the child's doctor or dentist to prescribe fluoride for children between the ages of 3 and 16 years. Children may also receive fluoride treatments at the dentist's office. Explain that fluoride mouth rinses are recommended for children over the age of 6 years. Parents can also buy toothpaste with fluoride in it.

Sealants

Explain what sealants are and why they are used. (Sealants are a plastic coating that is painted on the four permanent molars that come in when a child is about 6 or 7 years old, and the four molars that come in when a child is about 12 or 13 years old. They help to prevent cavities in the tops of the teeth.) Explain that sealants are usually applied at a dentist's office. The process does not hurt at all. The coating is usually painted on the tooth and given time to dry.

Nutrition

Present a visual of the food pyramid. Explain that for healthy bodies and healthy teeth, we need to eat foods from all the groups shown on the pyramid.

Reinforce that while a balanced diet is important in preventing cavities, tooth decay is also the result of what children eat, when, and how often. Explain that frequent snacking leaves food on the teeth longer, and thus is more apt to promote the decay process. For this reason, sugars and starches are best reserved for mealtime, when increased saliva production helps neutralize the acids produced by oral bacteria.

Discuss how research has shown that certain foods have "anti-cavity power"; that is, they reduce the acid exposure to the teeth. These foods are considered more dentally sound because they fight plaque and neutralize the bacteria that cause decay. They include:

- Cheese (e.g., Jack, Cheddar, Swiss)
- Raw fruits and vegetables
- Peanuts and cashews

Closure

(2–3 minutes, 5–10 minutes for questions)

- Restate the objectives in question form.
- Check attendees' knowledge and understanding of the concepts presented.
- If time permits, address any other questions attendees may have.

Lesson plan / COMMUNITY OUTREACH PROGRAM: PARENT EDUCATION MEETING

DATE _____ LOCATION _____

TIME (60–90 MINUTES) _____ CONTACT PERSON _____

PRESENTER(S) _____

Preparation in Classroom _____

_____

_____

_____

_____

_____

Anticipatory Planning _____

_____

_____

_____

_____

_____

_____

_____

_____

Review of Previous Objectives: _____

_____

_____

_____

_____

_____

_____

Three Specific Objectives:

1. _____

_____

2. _____

_____

3. _____

_____

Information to Be Presented Will Include:

(Topics) _____

_____

_____

_____

_____

_____

(Methods) _____

_____

_____

_____

_____

_____

(Lecture, demonstration, visual aids, group discussion) _____

_____

_____

_____

_____

_____

Guided Practice Activities _____

_____

_____

_____

_____

_____

Closure _____

_____

_____

_____

_____

_____

_____

Dental Health Fact Sheet

Food for Dental Health

Foods with sugar in them are very harmful to the teeth. It is important to limit the number of times a day sweet foods are eaten. Here are some ideas for good snack foods.

Nuts	Fresh fruits and vegetables
Sunflower seeds	Unsweetened juices
Popcorn	*Sugarless* gum, candy, soft drinks
Pretzels	Luncheon meats, beef jerky
Cheese	Leftover roast beef or chicken

Your Dentist

This school program does *not* take the place of regular dental checkups. It is important for your child to visit a dentist at least two times a year for checkups and/or dental repairs.

How You Can Help at Home

- Encourage your child to practice brushing and flossing at home every day (particularly before bed at night). It is important for you to watch the flossing and help your child so the gums will not be injured.
- As he or she learns to do a good job of tooth cleaning, ask your child to teach the rest of the family.

Children learn best by watching adults. Be a good role model; practice proper dental hygiene every day! Healthy teeth and gums . . . they can last a lifetime!

Dental Health Fact Sheet

"Smile in Style": Dental Disease Prevention Program

Dental disease can be prevented and your teeth *can* last a lifetime. Unfortunately, 8 out of 10 children have dental disease by the age of 9 years. More than 95 percent of adult Americans have dental disease, and 20 million Americans have lost all their teeth. All this can be prevented if everyone would learn and practice personal dental care!

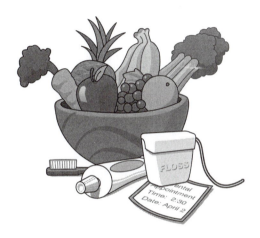

Your child's class is taking part in a "Smile in Style" Dental Disease Prevention Program. Students will learn ways of caring for their teeth and gums. Dental disease can be controlled if we practice daily care by brushing and flossing. To reinforce good dental habits, tooth cleaning and choosing good nutritious foods must be done at home *every* day in order to get the best results. Your participation is important.

Your Child Is Learning

- Teeth are important for eating, talking, happy smiles, and good health.
- There are two major dental diseases caused by germs living on and around the teeth: Tooth decay (cavities), and gum disease (gingivitis or pyorrhea).
- Some of the germs live in a sticky, hard-to-see film called plaque. Plaque forms on teeth every day.
  Plaque germs + Sugar (in *all* foods) + Acid = Tooth decay
  Germ plaque + Toxins (plaque waste product) = Gum disease
- Dental disease *can* be prevented. Help keep your teeth and gums healthy!
- Clean teeth daily with a toothbrush and dental floss.
- Eat fewer sweet foods that have sugar, especially for between-meal snacks.
- Help teeth fight decay by using some form of fluoride (fluoride toothpaste, fluoride tablets, topical applications by a dentist, or a weekly fluoride mouth rinse).

Information You Should Know

Always giving your child a bottle of milk or sweetened drink to take to bed can lead to serious tooth decay, known as baby bottle tooth decay. When a baby falls asleep with a bottle in his or her mouth, the milk or sweet liquid stays around the teeth. Germs and the sugar make acid which causes teeth to decay. Young children who walk around all day with a bottle in their mouth may also get many cavities for the same reason.

Your Child Is Learning to Use These Things to Clean His or Her Teeth

Toothbrush

A small toothbrush with soft, rounded bristles should be used to remove germ-filled plaque from teeth and gums.

- *Brush Biting Surfaces.* On the tops of teeth where you chew, the bristles should be pointed toward the grooves and moved gently back and forth.

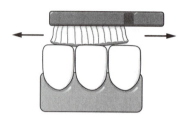

- *Vibrate Gently on Both Sides.* On cheek side and tongue side, bristles should be pointed toward the gum line and rocked gently in a short, wiggly motion. Children are cautioned not to scrub vigorously back and forth on these surfaces, as it can hurt the gums.

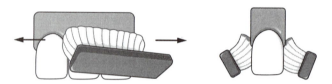

Dental Floss

Floss should be used to clean between the teeth where the toothbrush cannot reach. Most serious tooth decay and gum disease starts in these spaces. Each space has two tooth walls that must be cleaned. Start where the two teeth touch and clean all the way into the gum line space.

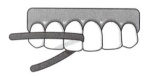

- Hold a 12- to 18-inch piece of floss by wrapping the ends around your middle fingers. Guide the floss between your teeth by holding it with your thumbs and first fingers.
- Curve the floss around one tooth and move it up and down gently several times, then curve it around the other tooth and move up and down before going on to the next space.

Fluoride Rinse and Fluoride Tablet Programs

Both programs are used in the classroom *by parental permission only.*

- Fluoride Rinse Program. The fluoride rinse is a solution that is used once a week. It is swished around in the mouth for a minute, and then spit out into a cup.
- Fluoride Tablet Program. The fluoride tablet is used daily after brushing. The tablet should be chewed for 30 seconds, swished for 30 seconds, and then swallowed.

Fluoride in either form strengthens teeth, providing protection against the cavity-causing agent, plaque.

Parent Meeting
presented by

_____

Help your child have healthy teeth.

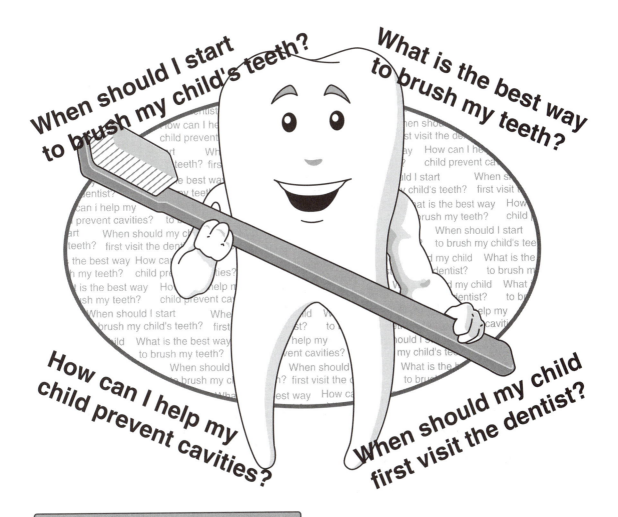

Learn the answers to these questions.
Date and Time:
Place:
Facilitator:

Free toothbrushes will be provided.

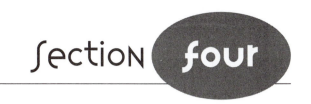
Integrating Dental Health Education Into the Classroom

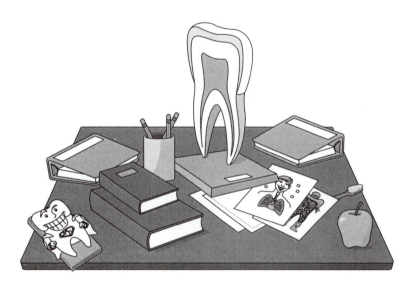

this section emphasizes ways to integrate dental health education into the regular academic curriculum and provides guidelines for developing visual aids that can assist you in your presentations. The goal is to develop informative activities and visuals that can be utilized by the classroom teacher and incorporated in classroom learning throughout the year. Dental health education is most effective when it is integrated into classroom activities and not fragmented or mentioned only when dental health educators are present.

Hints to Help Integrate the Dental Program Into the Academic Curriculum

Dental health concepts can be reinforced in several different areas of the elementary school curriculum. Following are suggested activities that can be utilized by teachers during creative writing, English, reading, social studies, math, and science/health portions of the curriculum.

—Arlene Globe, RDH

Creative Writings

- Have students write paragraphs on topics such as "My Life as a Tooth" or "My Life as a Loose Tooth."
- Have students create comic strips about teeth talking to each other that contain important messages about dental health.
- Have the class write a commercial for a new and exciting dental product. Students may create artwork to go with the commercial, and a song or jingle to describe the product.
- Have students write a paragraph on their feelings about their teeth.
- Have students design and write about inventions that might help care for teeth.
- Have the class design a dialogue between two or three teeth. Encourage students to ask questions such as, "What kind of tooth are you?, Where do you live and who are your neighbors?, and Does it cost much to care for you?"
- Have students write a scary story using characters such as the ghost-like Plaque and the evil Sweet Sugar. Illustrate the story.
- Valentine's Day, Christmas, Halloween, and Easter are times when we often overeat sweets. Ask children to write about a special holiday feast where something magical happened and good food choices were made.
- Divide students into groups. Have each group write a play about teeth. It can be fiction, nonfiction, or science fiction. Set aside one afternoon for the various performances. Supply healthy snacks as a treat.
- Research what's new in dentistry. Have students do a "News Bulletin" announcing the new discoveries.

English

- Have students write a poem about teeth.
- Ask students to interview their parents and about their dental experiences and then report back to the class.
- Create a dental spelling list (refer to the appendix listing of dental terms, and the glossary at the end of this book). Have the students write different sentences using each word.
- Ask students to write a letter to their dentist describing how they take care of their teeth and asking if there are any other things they can do.
- Ask students to write about the dental health professionals in their dental office, including who they are and what they do.

Reading

- Read one of the dental stories presented in Section Two. Have a discussion afterward. Have students draw or write about their favorite part of the story, or what they did or did not like about the story.
- Have students make up picture and word stories about teeth or another dental subject.
- Have students memorize a poem about teeth.

Social Studies

- Have students research the following topics: (1) how early settlers might have cared for their teeth, (2) the history of the toothbrush, (3) the history of dentistry, and (4) problems early settlers might have had with their teeth.
- Talk about changes in dental technology in the past 10 to 15 years. Then, have students write a report on these changes after interviewing their parents or a local dentist. Students should also be encouraged to use the school library for research.
- Have students make up their own laws about dental health and safety.
- Have students discuss how their eating patterns change when they're away from home (at camp, a relative's house, etc.). What kinds of things do they eat at camp? At their grandparents' house? When they're on vacation?
- Have students research the ways different people through the ages or from different countries have taken care of their teeth. The teacher may want to divide the class into groups and assign a different era or different country to each group.
- Have students design a map of a town with streets and public buildings. Have them place a real or fictional dental office on the map. Accompany the map with a short story about what goes on at a dental office or why we should go.

Math

- Create word problems for all grade levels using dental words or objects (see Fig. 4–4).
- Write a few logic and reasoning stories that contain math problems relating to dental facts, nutrition, or other related areas.
- Have students make an "acid attack chart" that lists every snack or meal eaten during the day. Add up the 20-minute periods after each snack or meal to get a total number indicating the amount of time acid is attacking the teeth. Make a graph of the information on the chart.

Science and Health*

- Make a poster of items that cause a lot of damage to the teeth. Try to design it so it sends a message without the use of words.
- Show students pictures of a healthy tooth and a decayed tooth. Ask students to create their own tooth out of cardboard or soap. Be sure to name all the parts of the tooth.
- Have students create a dental survey containing at least five questions relating to dental health. Tell them to ask at least 10 friends the questions, then bring the answers back to class and compare them. Have students write conclusions and recommendations from what they have learned.
- Make a hidden sugar display. (See the Section Two discussion of nutrition and healthy teeth.) Using common foods, ask students to add up the amount of sugar consumed in a day, a week, and a month.

*Prepared by the Office of Dental Health, Maine Department of Human Services.

- Science experiments are useful learning tools when working with students. Hands-on experiences have a lasting impact and illustrate concepts that are difficult to convey on paper. Four experiments that can be conducted in the classroom are described on the following pages.

Experiment 1: Spoiling apple

This experiment uses the decaying process of apples to illustrate dental decay.

Supplies

Two apples
Bowl

Directions

First, place an apple with a tiny spot on it in a bowl. The tiny spot will spread through the whole apple, which is similar to the manner in which decay progresses through the tooth. Cutting the apple in half will illustrate this process for students.

Next, place an apple with a small bruise spot touching an apple that is not bruised. In time, the apple that had no spot will have a decay spot on it. This illustrates how decay on one tooth will spread to the tooth that it is touching.

Experiment 2: Egg and vinegar

This experiment shows that acid weakens substances such as tooth enamel that contain calcium. It also shows that fluoride strengthens tooth enamel against acid, reinforcing the importance of brushing with fluoride toothpaste and receiving fluoride treatments regularly from the dental office.

Supplies

Two eggs (hard boiled)
A large pickle jar (empty)
White vinegar
A plastic food storage bag
Fluoride gel (obtained through your dentist or hygienists)

Directions

Take one egg and put it in the plastic bag containing the fluoride gel. Make sure the fluoride completely covers the entire eggshell. Leave the egg in fluoride overnight. Then take both eggs and place them in a jar containing vinegar. Examine the eggs every few hours. As the acid from the vinegar attacks the tooth, bubbles arise from it. Notice that one egg has more bubbles then the other. Leave the eggs overnight. Take both eggs out of the jar the next day and examine them. The shell of the egg that was placed in fluoride will be harder than that of the other egg.

Experiment 3: Effects of acid on teeth

This experiment illustrates how acid attacks tooth enamel, eventually leading to tooth decay.

Supplies

Extracted tooth
A small bottle
White vinegar

Directions

Place an undecayed tooth in a bottle containing vinegar. The stronger the vinegar and the longer the time, the greater the effect on the tooth. As the acid demineralizes the tooth, the enamel loses its translucency, turns a chalky opaque white, and becomes soft. Eventually, the tooth will become so soft you will be able to pierce it with a needle. These changes in the tooth are similar to the process by which a tooth decays in the mouth.

Experiment 4: Tooth in Coke

This experiment illustrates how foods containing sugar cause teeth to decay.

Supplies

A jar
A soft drink with high sugar content (e.g., Coca-Cola)
Extracted tooth

Directions

Pour some of the soft drink into a jar. Add the undecayed tooth. Let the tooth remain in the jar for 4 to 6 months. This is a good experiment to do at the beginning of the year. Students can note their observations throughout the year. Remove the tooth after 4 to 6 months. It should be soft and might crumble.

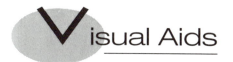

Visual Aids

Creating an Appropriate Visual Aid

Visual aids have several advantages in the classroom. They:

- Help the educator to present ideas exactly
- Appeal to more than one sense
- Broaden the learner's experience
- Are suitable for all ages
- Are effective when language barriers exist

The purpose of the visual aid is to: (1) assist the educator in attaining the objective of the lesson, and (2) improve the learning situation and make it meaningful. Among the various types of visual aids that can be used are:

- One-dimensional
- Two-dimensional
- Three-dimensional
- Audiovisual
- Creative plays or games

Examples of each of these types and ideas for using them in the classroom are presented below.

One-dimensional Visual Aids

One-dimensional visual aids include chalkboards or marker boards, charts, bulletin boards, flip-charts, projected aids, and duplicated aids.

Chalkboard/marker board

This board can be predrawn before the start of the lesson, or its use can be planned during the lesson or off-hand (suddenly you decide to draw, to explain a concept). It is available in most classrooms and can be especially effective when used with forethought.

Chart

A chart can be an effective aid, particularly when simple. When creating charts, focus on one idea, and make it graphic. Use color to distinguish different points or areas of the chart.
Charts can be used to:

- Present data (e.g., percentages of children with tooth decay)
- Provide a schematic representation of an idea (e.g., the decay process)
- Diagram activities or information
- Graph data

Bulletin board

A bulletin board is available in most classrooms and can be used to present a variety of ideas and materials. An effective bulletin-board display should project only one major idea. Use simple lettering and illustrations. The layout patterns can be symmetrical or diagonal.

Flip-chart

This is an inexpensive, permanent, and portable visual aid. Many types of preprinted flip-charts are available, including flash cards, stories, and charts; or create your own using a large tablet—flip through pre-drawn pages or draw as needed.

Projected aid

This category includes slides, single-concept films (usually between 2 and 4 minutes in length), and transparencies for use with an overhead projector. Slide programs have the advantages of being flexible, handy, and easily edited. Transparencies are easy to make.

Duplicated aids

This category includes any handouts or visuals made with a photocopier or other duplicating system.

Two-dimensional Visual Aids

Two-dimensional visual aids include flannel boards, Velcro boards, and self-stick lettering.

Felt board

A felt board is a relatively inexpensive aid that is particularly effective for small children, enabling them to replay the story or lesson. The size of the board should reflect the number of students or attendees. Be sure the board can be seen by all participants. Cover a large piece of light weight wood or foam board with felt. Cut-out characters can have velcro or sandpaper glued to the back so that they will stick on the board.

Lettering

Letters being displayed should be at least 2 inches in height. When using letters to convey a message, remember these tips:

- Make it **bold.**
- Make it BIG so all can see.
- Make it simple.

Three-dimensional Visual Aids

Educators can make use of a wide variety of three-dimensional aids, including:

- Cutout, cutaway, or cross-sectional models
- Working models
- Enlarged models
- Reduced models
- Transparent models
- Fantasized characters or dress (puppets, etc.)

The use of several such aids was suggested in the various lesson plans in Section Two. (See Fig. 4–1 and Fig. 4–3 for examples of instructional patterns.)

Audiovisual Aids

These include:

- Videocassette tapes
- Slide programs or films with audio scripts
- Compact disks, records, or tapes

All programs, tapes, or recordings should always be previewed before use. After presenting an audiovisual program, the educator should follow up with a discussion that stresses important points and reinforces learning.

Creative Play or Games

This educational strategy is one of the most effective instruments of human understanding and interaction. Children especially seem to enjoy the opportunity to act in plays and dramatizations of stories or events. Several such games and short plays were presented in Section Two.

Constructing a Large Tooth Model

Supplies

A 12- × 9- × 1-inch piece of Styrofoam (for teeth)
A 12- × 4.5- × 1-inch piece of Styrofoam (for gums)
A square of white felt
A half square of pink felt
Small pieces of red and black felt (for gingivitis and cavity)
Yarn (for floss)
Yellow or green cotton balls (for plaque)
Six, 2-inch nails
Glue and glue gun

Directions

1. Trace the tooth pattern from Figure 4–1A on the white felt.
2. Trace the gums pattern from Figure 4–1B on the pink felt.
3. Trace the tooth and the gum patterns onto the Styrofoam boards.
4. Cut out the Styrofoam using a serrated knife.
5. Glue the white felt to the Styrofoam teeth to create the tooth model. Let set.
6. Cut three, 1-inch wide by 4-inch long strips to use as a divider. Glue one strip on either side, and one in the middle of the Styrofoam teeth.
7. Glue the Styrofoam gums over the three dividers.
8. Dip the nails in glue. Push them from the back of model through the divider pieces and into the gums.
9. Glue the pink felt onto the Styrofoam gums.
10. Cut out red felt for the gums.
11. Cut out black felt for the cavity, following the pattern in Figure 4–1B.
12. Use the colored cotton balls for plaque.

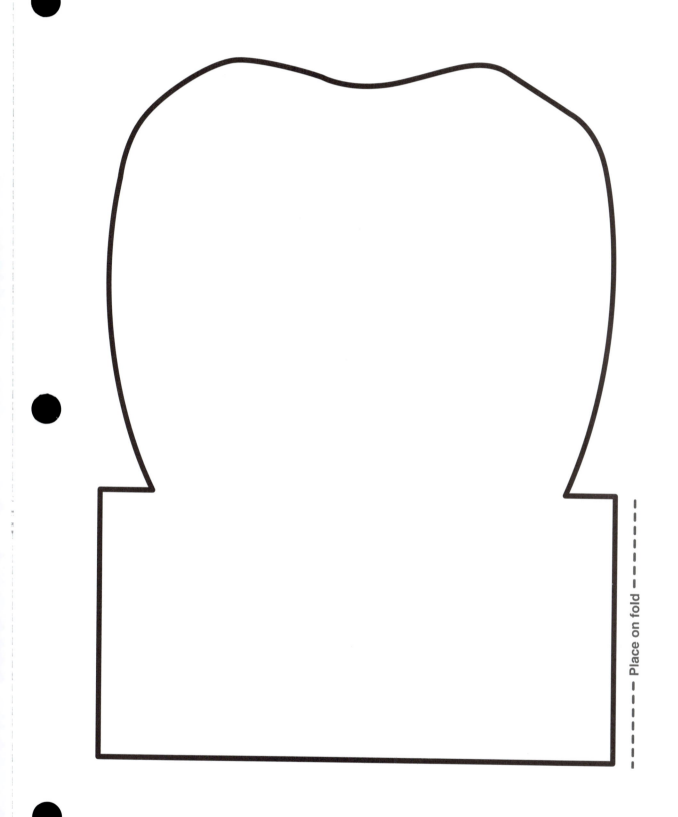

FIGURE 4–1A Large Tooth Pattern.

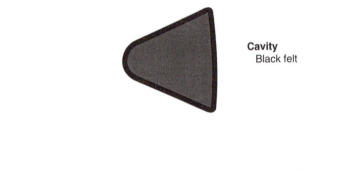

Cavity
Black felt

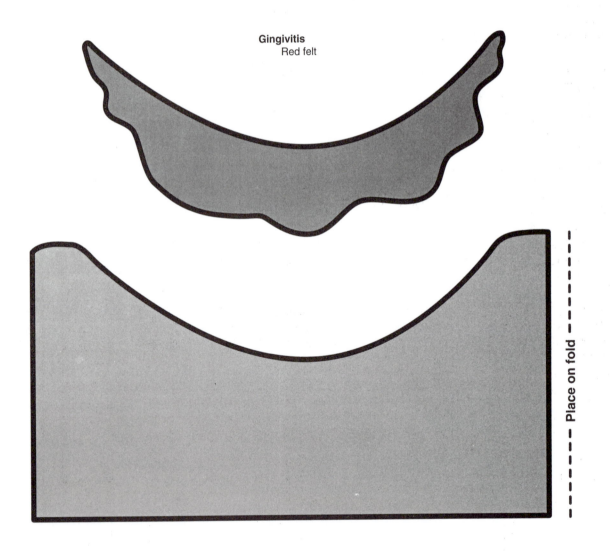

Gingivitis
Red felt

Place on fold

FIGURE 4–1B Large Tooth Pattern.

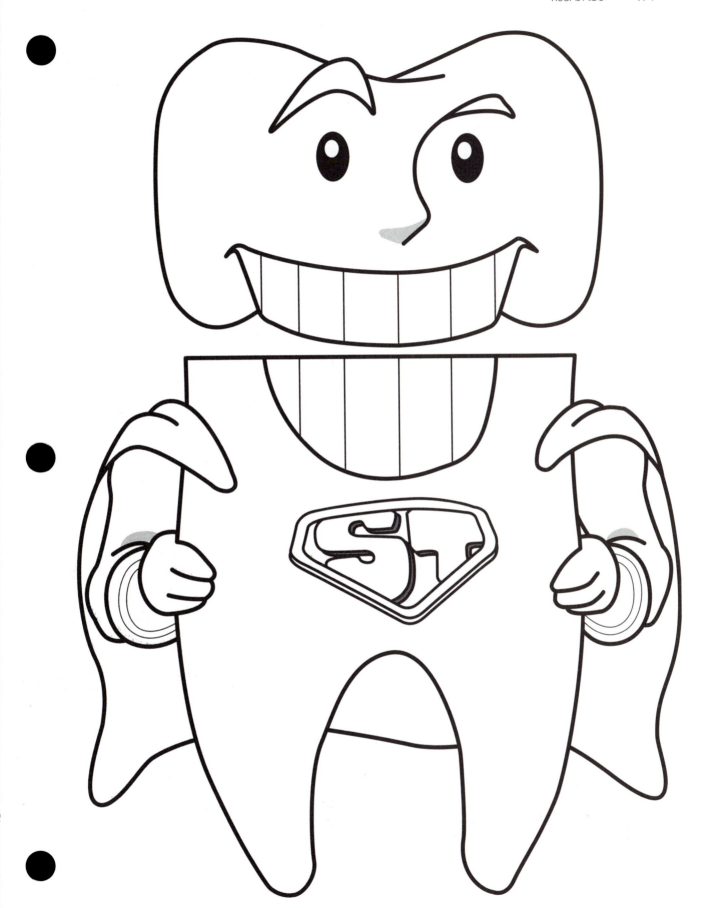

FIGURE 4–2A Super Tooth Model (front).

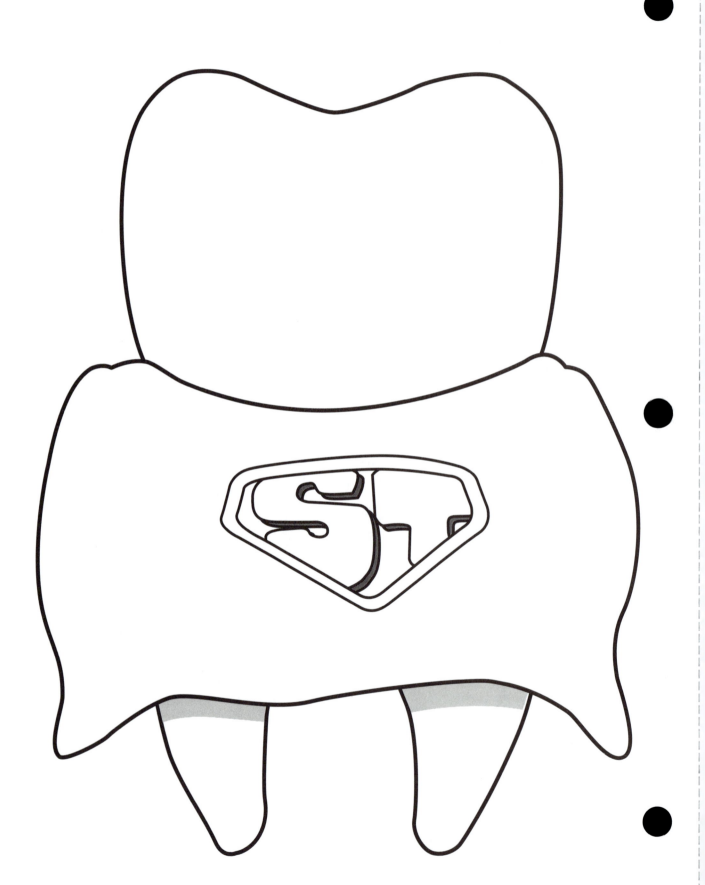

FIGURE 4–2B Super Tooth Model (back).

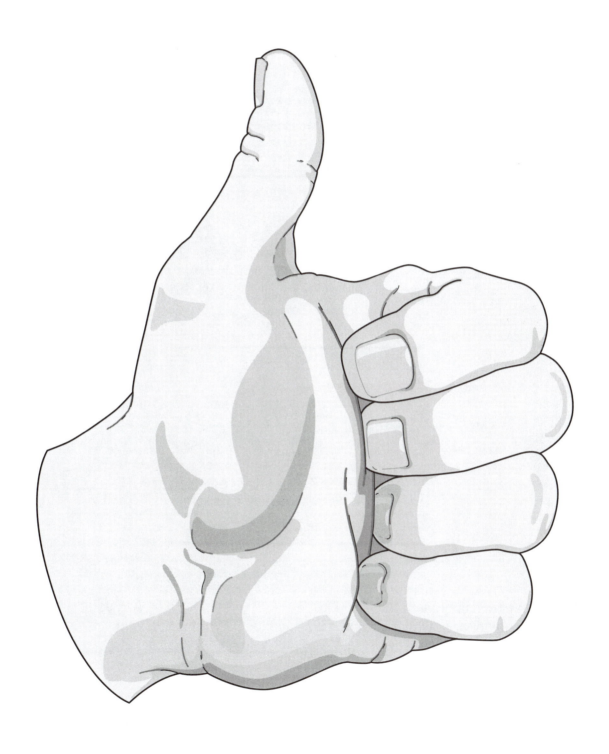

FIGURE 4–3 "Thumbs-up" model.

Tooth Math   NAME _____

1. 3 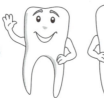 **+** 1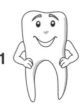

       = _____

2. 4 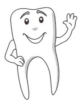 **+** 2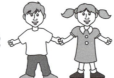

       = _____

3. 3 **+** 4

       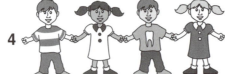

       = _____

4. How many teeth have you lost?_____Ask your
   neighbor how many teeth they have lost. What is the total
   number of teeth lost?_____.

5. Mary had 8 front teeth. 2 fell out. How many were left?_____

FIGURE 4–4 Tooth Math.

● Appendix: Additional Resources

$t$he seven dental health fact sheets included in this appendix were developed by the California Dental Association. Fact sheets are included on the following topics: Baby Bottle Tooth Decay; Dental Emergencies; Clean Teeth and Gums; Mouth Guards; Diet and Dental Health; If You Chew, Quit; and Sealants. Each fact sheet is presented first in English and then in Spanish translation. This information may be copied and distributed as needed. Also included in the appendix are a vocabulary list of dental terminology with definitions modified for children, and a resource guide to additional supplies.

Dental Health Fact Sheet

Baby Bottle Tooth Decay

Baby bottle tooth decay is a dental condition that can destroy the teeth of an infant or young child. The upper front teeth are the most susceptible to damage, but other teeth also may be affected.

What Causes Baby Bottle Tooth Decay?

Baby bottle tooth decay is caused by the frequent and long-term exposure of a child's teeth to liquids containing sugars. Among these liquids are milk, formula, fruit juice, sodas, and other sweetened drinks. The sugars in these liquids pool around the infant's teeth and gums, feeding the bacteria that cause plaque. Every time your child consumes a sugary liquid, acid attacks his or her teeth. After numerous attacks, tooth decay can occur, resulting in baby bottle tooth decay.

Parents and caregivers should be especially concerned with giving an infant a sugary drink at nap or night time. During sleep, the flow of saliva decreases, allowing the sugary liquids to pool around the child's teeth for an extended period of time.

How to Prevent Baby Bottle Tooth Decay

Parents sometimes do not realize that baby teeth are susceptible to decay as soon as they appear in the infant's mouth. By the time the decay is noticed, it may be too late to save the child's teeth. You can prevent this from happening to your child's teeth by knowing how to protect them.

- After each feeding, wipe the child's teeth and gums with a damp washcloth or small soft toothbrush to remove plaque. Begin brushing your child's teeth as soon as the first tooth erupts. Flossing should begin when all primary teeth have erupted, usually by age 2 or 2½.
- Never allow your child to fall asleep with a bottle containing a sweetened liquid.
- If your child refuses to fall asleep without a bottle, simply fill it with water and nothing else.
- If your local water supply does not contain enough decay-fighting fluoride, check with your dentist to see if your child should receive fluoride supplements.
- Start dental visits between 6 and 12 months of age.

How Serious Is Baby Bottle Tooth Decay?

Baby bottle tooth decay can cause painful toothaches, which can hinder eating. Severely decayed teeth can become infected and need to be extracted. If your child's teeth are infected or lost too early due to baby bottle tooth decay, your child may have some of these problems:

- Poor eating habits
- Speech problems
- Crooked teeth
- Damaged adult (permanent) teeth
- Yellow or brown adult (permanent) teeth

Keep your child happy and smiling by preventing baby bottle tooth decay.

Hoja de Datos Sobre la Salud Dental

La Podredumbre Dental de Biberón

La podredumbre dental de biberón es una condición dental que puede destruir los dientes de un infante o niño pequeño. Los dientes frontales de arriba son los más susceptibles al daño, pero otros dientes pueden también ser afectados.

¿Cuál es la Causa de la Podredumbre Dental de Biberón?

La podredumbre dental de biberón es causada por la frecuente y prolongada exposición de los dientes del niño a los líquidos que contienen azúcares. Entre estos líquidos se encuentran la leche, la fórmula, los jugos de fruta, los refrescos embotellados, y otros líquidos azucarados. Los azúcares en estos líquidos se estancan alrededor de los dientes y las encías del niño pequeño, alimentando las bacterias que causan la placa bacteriana. Cada vez que su niño consume un líquido azucarado, el ácido ataca sus dientes. Después de numerosos ataques, puede empezar la caries, y por fin la podredumbre dental de biberón.

Los padres y los que cuidan a los niños deben tomar especial cuidado en no dar al niño bebidas azucaradas ni a la hora de la siesta ni en la noche. Durante el sueño, el flujo de saliva se disminuye, permitiendo que los líquidos azucarados se estanquen alrededor de los dientes del niño por un tiempo prolongado.

Cómo Impedir la Podredumbre Dental de Biberón

Los padres a veces no se dan cuenta de que los dientes del bebé son susceptibles a la podredumbre tan pronto como aparecen en la boca del infante. En el momento en que la podredumbre se note, puede ser demasiado tarde salvar los dientes del niño. Usted puede evitar que esto suceda an los dientes de su niño sabiendo como protegerlos.

- Después de cada alimento, limpie los dientes y las encías del niño con un trapo húmedo o un cepillo de dientes pequeño y suave para quitar la placa bacteriana. Comience a cepillar los dientes de su niño tan pronto como el primer diente haga erupción. La limpieza con hilo dental debe comenzar cuando todos los dientes primarios hayan hecho erupción, usualmente a la edad de 2 ó 2½ años.
- Nunca permita que su niño se duerma con un biberón que contenga un líquido azucarado.
- Si su niño se resiste a dormir sin un biberón, simplemente llénelo con agua y nada más.
- Si su abastecimiento local de agua no contiene el fluoruro suficiente anti-podredumbre, consulte a su dentista para saber si su niño necesita recibir applicaciones de fluoruro.
- Comience las visitas al dentista entre los 6 y 12 meses.

¿Qué Tan Seria Es la Podredumbre Dental de Biberón?

La podredumbre dental de biberón puede causar dolores de dientes muy fuertes que no permiten comer. Los dientes severamente podridos pueden infectarse y necesitar ser extraídos. Si los dientes de su niño se infectan o se pierden a temprana edad debido a la podredumbre dental de biberón, su niño podría llegar a tener algunos de estos problemas:

- Hábitos alimenticios pobres
- Problemas de locución
- Dientes torcidos
- Dientes de adulto (permanentes) dañados
- Dientes de adulto (permanentes) amarillos o cafés

Mantenga a su niño feliz y sonriente protegiéndolo contra la podredumbre dental de biberón.

Dental Health Fact Sheet

Dental Emergencies

Injuries to the mouth may include teeth that are knocked out (evulsed), forced out of position (extruded), or broken (fractured). Sometimes lips, gums, or cheeks have cuts. Oral injuries are often painful, and should be treated by a dentist as soon as possible.

Evulsed Teeth

When a tooth is knocked out you should:

- Immediately call your dentist for an emergency appointment.
- Attempt to find the tooth.
- Gently rinse, but do not scrub the tooth to remove dirt or debris.
- Place the clean tooth in your mouth between the cheek and gum.
- Do not attempt to replace the tooth into the socket. This could cause further damage.
- Get to the dentist as soon as possible. If it is within 30 minutes of the injury, it may be possible to reimplant the tooth.
- If it is not possible to store the tooth in the mouth of the injured person, (e.g., young child), wrap the tooth in a clean cloth or gauze and immerse in milk.

Extruded Teeth

If the tooth is pushed out of place (inward or outward), it should be repositioned to its normal alignment with very light finger pressure. Do not force the tooth into the socket. Hold the tooth in place with a moist tissue or gauze. Again, it is vital that the injured individual be seen by a dentist within 30 minutes.

Fractured Teeth

How a fractured tooth is treated will depend on how badly it is broken. Regardless of the damage, treatment should always be determined by a dentist.

- **Minor Fracture.** Minor fractures can be smoothed by your dentist with a sandpaper disc or simply left alone. Another option is to restore the tooth with a composite restoration. In either case, you should treat the tooth with care for several days.
- **Moderate Fractures.** Moderate fractures include damage to the enamel, dentin, and/or pulp. If the pulp is not permanently damaged, the tooth may be restored with a full permanent crown. If pulpal damage does occur, further dental treatment will be required.
- **Severe Fracture.** Severe fractures often mean a traumatized tooth with a slim chance of recovery.

Injuries to the Soft Tissues of the Mouth

Injuries to the inside of the mouth include tears, puncture wounds, and lacerations to the cheek, lips, or tongue. The wound should be cleaned right away and the injured person taken to the emergency department for the necessary suturing and wound repair.

Bleeding from a tongue laceration can be reduced by pulling the tongue forward and using gauze to place pressure on the wound area.

Hoja de Datos Sobre la Salud Dental

Emergencias Dentales

Las lesiones en la boca pueden incluir dientes que se pierden por golpe (caídos), dientes forzados fuera de posición (movidos), o dientes rotos (fracturados). A veces los labios, las encías, o las mejillas tienen cortes, astas o úlceras. Las lesiones bucales son a menudo dolorosas, y deben ser tratadas por un dentista lo más pronto posible.

Dientes Caídos

Cuando un diente se ha caído usted debe:

- Llamar inmediatamente a su dentista y obtener una cita de emergencia.
- Intentar encontrar el diente.
- Enjuagar suavemente, pero sin restregar el diente, para quitarle cualquier residuo contaminante.
- Poner el diente limpio en su boca entre la mejilla y la encía.
- No intentar recolocar el diente en el agujero. Esto puede causar daño adicional.
- Ir al dentista lo antes posible. Dentro de los 30 minutos después de la lesión, podría ser posible reimplantar el diente.
- Si no es posible colocar el diente en la boca de la persona lesionada (eje., niño pequeño), envuelva el diente en un trapo limpio o gasa y sumérjalo en leche.

Diente Movido

Si el diente se ha empujado fuera de posición (hacia afuera o hacia adentro), debe ser recolocado en su alineación normal con una muy ligera presión del dedo. No lo fuerce hacia adentro del agujero. Mantenga el diente en su lugar con un papel sanitario mojado o gasa. Nuevamente, es forzoso que el individuo lesionado sea visto por un dentista antes de que pasen 30 minutos.

Diente Fracturado

El trata miento de un diente fracturado dependerá de la seriedad de la fractura. El tratamiento de cualquier fractura debe ser determinado por un dentista.

- **Fractura Menor.** Las fracturas menores pueden ser alisadas por su dentista con un disco de lija, o simplemente pueden quedarse sin tratamiento. Otra opción es la restauración del diente con un compuesto. En cualquier caso, el diente se debe tratar con cuidado por algunos días.
- **Fractura Moderada.** Las fracturas moderadas incluyen daño al esmalte, a la dentina, o a la pulpa. Si la pulpa no está permanentemente dañada, el diente puede ser restaurado por medio de una corona permanente. Si el daño a la pulpa ocurre, un tratamiento dental posterior será requerido.
- **Fractura Severa.** Las fracturas severas a menudo significan un trauma al diente con una probabilidad menor de recuperación.

Lesiones en los Tejidos Suaves de la Boca

La lesiones en el interior de la boca incluyen jalones, heridas punzantes, y laceraciones en la mejilla, los labios, o la lengua. La herida debe ser limpiada en seguida y la persona lesionada debe ser llevada a un departamento de emergencia para obtener las suturas y reparación necesarias de la herida.

El sangrado por una laceración de la lengua puede ser reducido al jalar la lengua hacia afuera y al usar una gasa para poner presión en el área de la herida.

Dental Health Fact Sheet

Clean Teeth and Gums

Having a clean mouth is important. In addition to being healthier, it gives you fresh breath and a nicer smile.

When you eat, bits of food, some too small for you to see, remain in your mouth. They feed bacteria that grow in a sticky film on your teeth. This film, called plaque, is the main cause of tooth decay and gum disease.

Why Brush?

Brushing your teeth after meals and between-meal snacks not only gets rid of the food particles that you can see, it removes plaque from your teeth. Using a fluoride toothpaste is important because the fluoride can help kill bacteria, as well as make your teeth stronger.

Ask your dentist to recommend the best toothbrush for you. Generally, a brush with soft, end-rounded or polished bristles is less likely to injure gum tissue. The size and shape of the brush should allow you to reach every tooth. Children may need smaller brushes than those designed for adults. Remember: Worn-out toothbrushes cannot properly clean your teeth and may injure your gums. Toothbrushes should be replaced every 3 or 4 months.

Why Floss?

Flossing removes plaque and food particles from between teeth and under the gum line; areas your toothbrush cannot reach. Because tooth decay and periodontal disease often start in these areas, it is important to clean them thoroughly on a daily basis.

Flossing is a skill that needs to be learned. Do not be discouraged if you find it difficult at first. With practice, you will find that flossing takes only a few minutes of your time each day.

What About Mouth Rinses and Mouthwashes?

If used as directed, in addition to brushing and flossing, mouth rinses and mouthwashes can help to prevent tooth decay.

How Often Should I See My Dentist?

If possible, you should visit your dentist every 6 months for a preventive check and cleaning. Infants should see a dentist at about 12 months of age.

Hoja de Datos Sobre la Salud Dental

Dientes y Encías Limpios

Es importante mantener una boca limpia. Además de ser saludable, le da un aliento fresco y una sonrisa más agradable.

Cuando come, pedazos de comida, algunos demasiado pequeños para ser vistos, permanecen en la boca. Estos alimentan a las bacterias que crecen en forma de película pegajosa en sus dientes. Esta capa, llamada placa bacteriana, es la causa principal de la podredumbre de los dientes y de la enfermedad de las encías.

¿Por Qué Cepillarse los Dientes?

Cepillarse los dientes después de las comidas y bocadillos entre comidas no sólo les quita las partículas de comida que usted puede ver, sino que también les quita la placa bacteriana. Usar una pasta con fluoruro es importante porque el fluoruro puede matar las bacterias, así como fortalecer sus dientes.

Pida a su dentista que le recomiende el cepillo de dientes más adecuado para usted. Generalmente, un cepillo con cerdas suaves y redondeadas o pulidas tiene menos posibilidad de dañar el tejido de las encías. El tamaño y forma del cepillo debe permitirle alcanzar cada diente. Los niños podrían necesitar cepillos más pequeños que los diseñados para adultos. Recuerde: Los cepillos de dientes desgastados no pueden limpiar propiamente los dientes y pueden dañar las encías. Los cepillos de dientes deben reemplazarse cada 3 o 4 meses.

¿Por Qué Limpiarse los Dientes con Hilo Dental?

Limpiar los dientes con hilo dental quita la placa bacteriana y las partículas de comida de entre los dientes y de debajo de la base de las encías, áreas que su cepillo de dientes no alcanza. Debido a que la podredumbre dental y la enfermedad de las encías frecuentemente empiezan en estas áreas, es importante limpiarlas diariamente.

La limpieza con hilo dental es una habilidad que necesita aprenderse. No se desanime si lo encuentra difícil en un principio. Con práctica, descubrirá que la limpieza con hilo dental toma sólo unos cuantos minutos de su tiempo cada día.

¿Qué de los Limpiadores y Enjuagues Bucales?

Si se usan de acuerdo con las instrucciones, además de cepillarse y limpiarse los dientes con hilo dental, los limpiadores y enjuagues bucales pueden ayudar a impedir la podredumbre dental.

¿Qué Tan Frecuentemente Debo Ver a Mi Dentista?

De ser posible, usted debe visitar a su dentista cada 6 meses para un examen preventivo y limpieza. Los niños deben ver al dentista a partir de los 12 meses de edad.

Dental Health Fact Sheet

Mouth Guards

Don't be the victim of a preventable injury: Wear a mouth guard. While mouth guards are not mandatory equipment in all sports, their worth is indisputable. Dentists see many oral and facial injuries that might have been prevented by the use of a mouth guard.

Facial injuries in nearly every sport can result in damage to teeth, lips, cheeks, and tongue. Mouth guards cushion blows to the face and neck. A mouth guard should be part of every athlete's gear, no matter the sport. It's better to play it safe than face a devastating and painful oral injury.

Even adults are not free from the dangers of mouth injuries. Dentists treat many trauma injuries in weekend athletes. Whatever your age or sport, mouth guards are an important part of sports safety and your exercise routine. Do what you can to protect your smile and preserve your health.

Dos and Don'ts

- Do wear a mouth guard at all times when playing sports.
- Do inform yourself about the most common oral injuries.
- Do wear a mouth guard custom-fitted by your dentist, especially if you wear fixed dental appliances such as braces or bridgework.
- Do not wear removable appliances (retainers, bridge, or complete or partial dentures) when playing sports.

What Are Your Choices?

There are three types of mouth guards: custom-made, mouth-formed, and ready-made. Custom-made mouth guards are professionally designed by your dentist from a cast model of your teeth. Because they are designed to cover all back teeth and cushion the entire jaw, they can prevent concussions caused by blows to the chin. Custom guards may be slightly more expensive than commercially produced mouthpieces, but they offer the best possible fit and protection. They are more secure in the mouth and do not interfere with speech or breathing. Calling plays or formations, for instance, will not be impeded by custom guards.

Mouth-formed guards, also called "boil and bite," should also be fitted by your dentist. This is generally done by shaping a soft preformed guard to the contours of the teeth and allowing it to harden. However, these devices are difficult to design for athletes who wear braces and can become brittle after prolonged use.

Ready-made, commercial mouth guards can be purchased at most sporting goods stores and are made of rubber or polyvinyl. They are the least expensive but also the least effective.

Keep your mouth guard in top shape by rinsing it with water or mouthwash after each use and allowing it to air-dry. With proper care, it should last the length of a season or longer.

Hoja de Datos Sobre la Salud Dental

Los Protectores Bucales

No sea víctima de una lesión previsible: Lleve un protector bucal. Aunque los protectores bucales no sean equipo obligatorio en todos los deportes, su mérito no tiene disputa. Los dentistas ven muchas lesiones bucales y faciales que hubieran podido preverse con un protector bucal.

Las lesiones faciales en casi todo deporte pueden lastimar los dientes, los labios, las mejillas, y la lengua. Los protectores bucales amortiguan los golpes en la cara y la nuca. Un protector bucal debe formar parte del equipo de todo atleta, en cualquier deporte. Mas vale jugar con seguridad que sufrir una lesión bucal devastadora y dolorosa.

Aún los adultos corren el riesgo de sufrir lesiones bucales. Los dentistas tratan muchas lesiones traumáticas de atletas de fin de semana. A cualquier edad y en cualquier deporte los protectores bucales son importantes para la sequridad deportiva y en su rutina de ejercicio. Haga lo posible por proteger la sonrisa y preservar la salud.

Lo Que Hacer y No Hacer

- Lleve un protector bucal siempre al practicar los deportes.
- Infórmese sobre las lesiones bucales más comunes.
- Lleve un protector bucal moldeado a la medida por su dentista, sobre todo si lleva aparatos dentales fijos como frenos o puentes.
- No lleve aparatos movibles (retenedores, puentes, o dentaduras completas o parciales) cuando practique los deportes.

¿Cuáles Son Sus Alternativas?

Existen tres tipos de protector bucal: a la medida, conformados directamente a la detadura, y prefabricados. Los protectores bucales a la medida son diseñados profesionalmente por su dentista a partir de una forma moldeada de su dentadura. Ya que están diseñados para cubrir todos los dientes traseros y para ayudar a amortiguar completamente la mandíbula, pueden prevenir las concusiones causadas por golpes en la barbilla. Los protectores bucales a la medida pueden ser un poco más caros que aquellas piezas bucales producidas comercialmente, pero ofrecen el mejor ajuste y protección posibles. Se ajustan con más seguridad en la boca y no interfieren con el habla o la respiración. El ordenar jugadas y formaciones, por ejemplo, no será impedido por los protectores bucales a la medida.

Los protectores moldeados directo sobre la dentadura deben también ser ajustados por su dentista. Estos protectores se hacen generalmente con un protector suave que se conforma a la dentadura y se deja endurecer. Sin embargo, estas piezas son difíciles de diseñar para atletas que usan frenos y pueden quedar quebradizas después del uso prolongado.

Los protectores bucales comerciales prefabricados pueden conseguirse en la mayoría de las tiendas de deportes, y son hechos de hule o polivinilo. Son los menos caros, pero también los menos efectivos.

Conserve su protector bucal en óptinas condicines al enjuagarlo con agua o enjuague bucal después de cada uso y dejarlo secar al aire. Con el cuidado apropiado, un protector bucal debe durar una temporada o más.

Dental Health Fact Sheet

Diet and Dental Health

You know that what you eat can make a difference in the way you feel and perform. That is why you should try to choose foods that will help your body stay strong and healthy. But did you know that your choice of foods and your eating patterns also may affect your dental health?

How Does Diet Affect Dental Health?

If your diet is low in certain nutrients, it may be harder for the tissues of your mouth to resist infection. This may be a contributing factor to periodontal (gum) disease, the main cause of tooth loss in adults. Although poor nutrition does not actually cause periodontal disease, many researchers believe that the disease progresses faster and is more severe in patients whose diet does not supply the necessary nutrients.

To make sure that you are getting enough nutrients for good general and oral health, you should choose foods from the four basic food groups: fruits and vegetables; breads and cereals; milk and dairy products; and meat, fish, and eggs. When you do snack, avoid soft, sweet, sticky foods, such as cakes, candy, and dried fruits, that cling to your teeth and promote tooth decay. Instead, choose dentally healthy foods such as nuts, raw vegetables, plain yogurt, cheese, popcorn, and sugarless gum or candy. To have a diet that promotes dental health, you must develop sensible eating habits.

How Can I Get Enough Fluoride?

If you and your family have a balanced diet, you will get all the nutrients you need for good dental health, with one possible exception—fluoride. Fluoride is vital for strong, decay-resistant teeth. If there is not enough fluoride in your community water supply, the level of fluoride can be adjusted to the right amount for good dental health (about one part fluoride per million parts water). If your drinking water is not fluoridated, ask your dentist how you can get the fluoride you need.

Fluoride toothpastes and mouth rinses that carry the seal of the American Dental Association's Council on Dental Therapeutics have been proven effective in helping prevent dental decay. However, they do not contribute to your dietary fluoride.

Together, a balanced diet, daily use of fluoride, brushing and flossing, and sensible eating habits, can reduce the risk of or even prevent dental disease.

Hoja de Datos Sobre la Salud Dental

Salud Dental y Dieta

Usted sabe que lo que come puede hacer la diferencia en cuanto a cómo se siente y cómo rinde. Por eso debe tratar de seleccionar alimentos que ayudarán a que su cuerpo se mantenga fuerte y sano. Pero, ¿sabía usted que la selección de alimentos y sus patrones alimienticios podrían también afectar su salud dental?

¿Cómo la Dieta Afecta la Salud Dental?

Si su dieta es baja en ciertos nutrimentos, podría ser más difícil para los tejidos de su boca resistir las infecciones. Esto podría ser un factor contribuyente pare la enfermedad de las encías, la causa principal de la pérdida de dientes en los adultos. A pesar de que de hecho la nutrición pobre no causa la enfermedad de las encías, muchos investigadores creen que la enfermedad progresa más rápidamente y es más severa en pacientes cuya dieta no suple los nutrimentos necesarios.

Para asegurarse de obtener suficientes nutrimentos pare tener buena salud general y bucal, debe seleccionar alimentos de los cuatro grupos alimenticios básicos: frutas y vegetales; panes y cereales; leche y productos lácteos; y carne, pescado, y huevos. Cuando come entre comidas, evite los alimentos suaves, dulces, y pegajosas, como los pasteles, dulces, y frutas secas, que se pegan a los dientes y pueden causar la caries. Es mejor escoger alimentos saludables para los dientes como nueces, verduras crudas, yogurt puro, queso, rosetas de maíz, y goma de mascar o dulces sin azúcar. Para tener una dieta propicia para la salud dental, usted debe desarrollar buenos hábitos alimenticios.

¿Cómo Puedo Obtener Suficiente Fluoruro?

Si usted y su familia tienen una dieta balanceada, obtendrán todos los nutrimentos que necesitan para una buena salud dental, con una posible excepción—el fluoruro. El fluoruro es esencial para una dentadura fuerte y resistente a las caries. Si no hay suficiente fluoruro en el abastecimiento de agua de su comunidad, el nivel de fluoruro puede ser ajustado a la cantidad correcta para una buena salud dental (una parte de fluoruro por un millón de partes de agua, aproximadamente). Si el agua potable que bebe no tiene fluoruro, pregunte a su dentista como puede obtener el fluoruro que necesita.

Las pastas y enjuagues bucales con fluoruro que llevan el sello del Consejo de la Asociación Dental Americana de Terapéutica Dental (American Dental Association's Council on Dental Therapeutics) se han probado efectivas en la ayuda a la prevención de la podredumbre dental. Sin embargo, no cumplen el requisito de fluoruro en la dieta.

En conjunto, una dieta balanceada, el uso diario de fluoruro, el cepillarse y limpiarse los dientes con hilo dental, y los buenos hábitos alimenticios, pueden reducir el riesgo de enfermedades dentales y aún prevenirlas.

Dental Health Fact Sheet

If You Chew, Quit

Smokeless tobacco use in the United States continues to increase each year. It may be smokeless, but it isn't harmless. Why should you care? Keep reading.

Smokeless Tobacco

- **Tooth Abrasion.** Grit and sand in smokeless tobacco products scratches teeth and wears away the hard surface or enamel. Premature loss of tooth enamel can cause added sensitivity and may require corrective treatment.
- **Gum Recession.** Constant irritation to the spot in the mouth where a small wad of chewing tobacco is placed can result in permanent damage to periodontal tissue. It also can damage the supporting bone structure. The injured gums pull away from the teeth, exposing root surfaces and leaving teeth sensitive to heat and cold. Erosion of critical bone support leads to loosened teeth that can be permanently lost.
- **Increased Tooth Decay.** Sugar is added to smokeless tobacco during the curing and processing to improve its taste. The sugar reacts with bacteria found naturally in the mouth, causing an acid reaction, which leads to decay.
- **Tooth Discoloration and Bad Breath.** Common traits of long-term smokeless tobacco users are stained teeth and bad breath. Moreover, the habit of continually spitting can be both unsightly and offensive.
- **Nicotine Dependence.** Nicotine blood levels achieved by smokeless tobacco use are similar to those from cigarette smoking. Nicotine addiction can lead to an artificially increased heart rate and blood pressure. In addition, it can constrict the blood vessels that are necessary to carry oxygen-rich blood throughout the body. Athletic performance and endurance levels are decreased by this reaction.
- **Unhealthy Eating Habits.** Chewing tobacco lessens a person's sense of taste and ability to smell. As a result, users tend to eat more salty and sweet foods, both of which are harmful if consumed in excess.
- **Oral Cancer.** With the practice of "chewing" and "dipping," tobacco and its irritating juices are left in contact with gums, cheeks, and/or lips for prolonged periods of time. This can result in a condition called leukoplakia. Leukoplakia appears either as a smooth, white patch or as leathery-looking wrinkled skin. It results in cancer in 3 percent to 5 percent of all cases.
- **Other Cancers.** All forms of smokeless tobacco contain high concentrations of cancer-causing agents. These substances subject users to an increased cancer risk not only of the oral cavity, but also of the pharynx, larynx, and esophagus.
- **Danger Signs.** If you use smokeless tobacco, or have in the past, you should be on the lookout for some of these early signs of oral cancer:
  - A sore that does not heal
  - A lump or white patch
  - A prolonged sore throat
  - Difficulty in chewing
  - Restricted movement of the tongue or jaws
  - A feeling of something in the throat

Pain is rarely an early symptom. For this reason, all tobacco users need regular dental checkups.

Hoja de Datos Sobre la Salud Dental

Si Used lo Mastica, Deje de Hacerlo

El uso de tabaco para masticar en los Estados Unidos continúa incrementándose cada año. Es cierto que no se fuma, pero no es inofensivo. ¿Por qué debe preocuparlo? Siga leyendo.

Tabaco Para Masticar

- **Raspadura de los Dientes.** Las partículas ásperas y la arenilla de los productos de tabaco para masticar raspan los dientes y desgastan la superficie dura o esmalte dental. La pérdida prematura del esmalte dental puede aumentar la sensibilidad dental y podría requerir un tratamiento correctivo.
- **Recesión de las Encías.** La constante irritación del lugar de la boca donde se acomoda la pequeña masa de tabaco para masticar puede resultar en daño permanente en el tejido periodontal. También puede dañar la estructura ósea de soporte. Las encías lesionadas se alejan del diente, exponiendo las superficies de la raíz y dejando el diente sensible al calor y al frío. El desgaste del soporte esencial de hueso puede ocasionar aflojamiento y, últimamente, la pérdida del diente.
- **Caries Incrementada de los Dientes.** Al tabaco para masticar se le agrega azúcar durante su curado y procesado para mejorar su sabor. El azúcar reacciona con las bacterias que se encuentran naturalmente en la boca, causando una reacción ácida, que provoca las caries.
- **Decoloración Dental y Mal Aliento.** Las características comunes de los habituados al tabaco para masticar son los dientes decolorados y el mal aliento. Además, el hábito de escupir contínuamente puede ofender tanto a la vista como a las buenas costumbres.
- **Dependencia a la Nicotina.** El nivel de nicotina en la sangre es parecida en el que mastica tabaco y el que fuma cigarrillos. La adicción a la nicotina puede ocasionar un incremento crónico en el bombeo de sangre por el corazón y un aumento en la presión arterial. Además, puede comprimir los vasos sanguíneos que transportan sangre rica en oxígeno a través del cuerpo. El rendimiento atlético y los niveles de resistencia disminuyen por esta reacción.
- **Hábitos Alimenticios no Saludables.** El masticar tabaco mengua el sentido del gusto y la capacidad de olfato de una persona. Como resultado, los usuarios tienden a comer alimentos más salados y dulces, los que son perniciosos si se consumen en exceso.
- **Cáncer Bucal.** El tabaco y sus jugos irritantes se quedan en contacto con las encías, las mejillas, y los labios por un tiempo prolongado. Esto puede ocasionar una condición llamada leucoplaquia. La leucoplaquia aparece ya sea en forma de parche blanco y suave o de arruga correosa. Degenera en cáncer del 3 al 5 por ciento de los casos.
- **Otros Tipos de Cáncer.** Todas las formas de tabaco para masticar contienen altas concentraciones de agentes causantes de cáncer. Estas sustancias someten a los usuarios a riesgos crecientes de cáncer no sólo de la cavidad bucal, sino también de la faringe, la laringe, y del esófago.
- **Señales de Peligro.** Si usted hace usa el tabaco para masticar, o lo ha hecho en el pasado, debe de estar pendiente de algunas de estas primeras señales de cáncer bucal:
  - Una llaga que no se cura
  - Un bulto o parche blanco
  - Un dolor de garganta prolongado
  - Dificultad al masticar
  - Movimiento restringido de la lengua o de las mandíbulas
  - La sensación de tener algo en la garganta

El dolor es raramente un síntoma temprano. Por esta razón, todo usuario de tabaco necesita exámenes dentales regulares.

Dental Health Fact Sheet

Sealants

With the help of your dentist, preventing tooth decay can become even easier. You may already be aware that daily brushing and flossing are the most important weapons against the formation of plaque, the primary cause of cavities. To supplement your regular routine of brushing and flossing, your dentist can apply a coat of plastic material—called a sealant—on the top, or biting, surfaces of your teeth. This plastic coating creates a barrier between your teeth and the decay-causing bacteria that live in plaque.

What Is Plaque and Why Does It Cause Cavities?

As you or your children eat and drink during the day, the food in your mouth combines with bacteria to produce a sticky film called plaque that attaches on and in between tooth surfaces (tooth enamel). Plaque often is found on the chewing surfaces of the back teeth, from which it is difficult to remove by brushing and flossing alone. If plaque is not removed regularly from your teeth, it can produce acids which will attack the tooth enamel and create pits or holes (cavities) in the tooth. This is tooth decay.

How Can Sealants Help Prevent Cavities?

Coating your teeth with a slippery plastic material makes it harder for plaque to stick to the tiny grooves on the biting surfaces of the teeth—reducing the risk of forming cavities and tooth decay.

Is It Difficult to Apply Sealants?

No. Your dentist may use a special instrument to apply the plastic sealant on your teeth. Most often, it is a painless treatment that lasts for many months.

Who Should Get Sealants?

Sealants are most effective in reducing cavities in children with newly formed permanent teeth. They are useful in cutting down formation of decay in adult teeth, as well. An application of sealants is a preventive measure to keep teeth healthy. It is an effective way to reduce the need for fillings and more expensive treatment that may be required to repair the damage from cavities, so sealants can also save you money.

Ask your dentist whether sealants would be an appropriate treatment for you and your children.

Hoja de Datos Sobre la Salud Dental

Los Selladores

Con la ayuda de su dentista, resultará todavía más fácil proteger contra la podredumbre dental. Usted ya sabrá que el cepillarse los dientes y limpiarse con hilo dental diariamente son las armas más importantes contra la formación de la placa bacteriana, que es la causa principal de las caries. Para complimentar la rutina regular de cepillarse los dientes y limpiarse con hilo dental, su dentista puede aplicar una capa de material plástico—llamado sellador—sobre las superficies de los dientes. Esta capa de plástico crea una barrera entre sus dientes y las bacterias que causan las caries y que viven en la placa bacteriana.

¿Qué Es la Placa Bacteriana y Por Qué Causa Caries?

Cuando usted o sus niños comen o beben durante el día, la comida en su boca se combina con las bacterias para formar una película pegajosa que se llama placa bacteriana, la cual se deposita encima y entre los dientes. La placa se encuentra a menudo sobre la superficie de las muelas traseras que se usan para masticar, de donde es difícil quitarla con sólo cepillarse y limpiarse con hilo dental. Si la placa no se quita regularmente de los dientes, puede producir ácidos que atacarán el esmalte y darán lugar a la formación de cavidades (caries) en el diente. Esto es la podredumbre dental.

¿Cómo Pueden los Selladores Prevenir las Caries?

Al recubrir sus dientes con un material plástico resbaloso es más difícil que la placa se pegue a los pequeños surcos de las superficies para masticar de los dientes—reduciendo así el riesgo de que se formen caries y la podredumbre dental.

¿Es Difícil Aplicar Selladores?

No. Su dentista puede usar un instrumento especial para aplicar el sellador plástico sobre sus dientes. La mayoría de las veces es un tratamiento que no duele y que dura muchos meses.

¿Quién Debe Usar Selladores?

Los selladores dan los mejores resultados para reducir las caries en niños con dientes permanentes recién formados. También son útiles para reducir la formación de caries en los adultos. La aplicación de un sellador es una medida preventiva para mantener su dentadura sana. Es una manera eficaz de reducir la necesidad de empastes y de tratamientos más caros que podrían ser necesarios para reparar los daños producidos por las caries, y por lo tanto, los selladores le pueden ahorrar dinero.

Pregúntele a su dentista si los selladores constituyen un tratamiento adecuado para usted y sus niños.

tooth Talk Dental Vocabulary

Table A–1 presents several common dental terms, accompanied by phrases that can be used when explaining these words to children or adult learners. This information can be given to the classroom teacher to incorporate as spelling words or given to the students to use when writing creative dental stories. Words and phrases can also be incorporated into year-end review lesson games and activities (such as matching word and description).

Table A–1 Tooth Talk Dental Vocabulary for Children and Adults

Tooth Talk	Children	Adults
Abscess	Bubble on the gums	Gum, boil, localized infection
Acid	Liquid that burns holes in teeth, tooth dissolver, eats holes in teeth	Liquid that burns holes
Air–water syringe	Wind–water gun, air gun, squirt gun	Spray used in the dental office to rinse off the tooth and gums
Amalgam/alloy	Silver star, silver filling	Silver filling
Aspirator	Little straw, vacuum cleaner	Used to remove water and debris from the mouth.
Blood	Red, hem, pink, RBCs	Blood
Bone loss	Bone disappears	Bone dissolves, is destroyed, is infected and loss of tooth support
Calculus	Tooth rocks, barnacles, coral	Calcified plaque, tartar, hard deposits, barnacles, or stones.
Cavity, caries	Hole in tooth, sick tooth, rotten, cave in tooth	Hole in tooth from decay
Curet/scaler	Little toothpick to clean your teeth, tooth cleaner, little spoon	Dental instrument to clean your teeth
Curettage		Removes the diseased or infected tissue inside the tooth and around the gum
Decay	Caused by the plaque + sugar = acid on healthy tooth = decay = cavities	
Dental floss	Like a piece of thread, string used to clean in between the teeth	Waxed, unwaxed, or tape, thin string used to remove plaque in between the teeth
Disclosing agent	Food coloring dye—shows if teeth are clean or dirty, red paint	Liquid or tablet, used for coloring the plaque, to make it visible
Explorer	Like a toothpick, tooth counter, tooth feeler	Dental instrument, used to check the teeth for cavities and calculus
Fluoride	Tooth hardener, shield, vitamins, added to toothpaste to make teeth strong	Substance that makes the tooth harder and stronger
Gingiva	Gums, skin around the tooth	
Gingivitis	Weak, soft, sick gums and unhealthy, puffy, red gums	A disease condition of the gums, infection, swelling

(continued)

Table A–1 Tooth Talk Dental Vocabulary for Children and Adults (continued)

Tooth Talk	Children	Adults
Hurt/pain	Bother, uncomfortable	
Head and neck exam		Checking to make sure glands and tissues are normal (healthy)
Plaque	Sticky, film of invisible bacteria, germs, sugar bugs that cause holes in your teeth	Film or colonies of invisible bacteria
Pocket		Infection on the inside of the gums, hole between the tooth and gums
Prophy angle	Electric toothbrush used in a dental office to clean the tooth	Used with a rubber cup in the dental office to polish the teeth after cleaning
Periodontitis		Infection of gums and bone, puss, bleeding, advanced gingivitis
Recession		Shrinkage of gums, gums pull away from tooth
Root planing		Smooth the root surface, clean the root surfaces
Slow speed	Air whistle, Mr. Bumpy	
Saliva Ejector	Mr. Slurpy, Mr. Thirsty	
Stainless steel crown	Silver hat, tooth hat	
Sulcus	Space around the tooth, between the tooth and gums	Cuff around tooth, little flap, space between the tooth and gums
Topical	Flavored jelly stick	
X-ray	Black and white picture of your teeth	Radiographs, dental films of your teeth
Xylocaine	Sleepy juice	Anesthesia

Courtesy of Diane Melrose, RDH, BS.

dental Health Educational Resources

Table A–2 is a detailed listing of several different types of resources that may be useful to the dental health educator who is planning presentations for children in grades K–6. Since prices are subject to change, it is best if you contact each source to obtain their latest catalog.

Table A–2   Selected Dental Health Educational Resources

Item and Description	Source
Flipchart	
Baby Bottle Tooth Decay Prevention Pictures and script, for individual or group discussion	American Dental Association 211 E. Chicago Ave. Chicago, IL 60611-2678 (800)947–4746 Fax: (312)440–3542
Toothtalk (1975) Grades K–3, pictures and script, lesson activities	American Society of Dentistry for Children 211 E. Chicago Ave. Chicago, IL 60611 (800)947–4746
Videos	
Parents Helping Parents A 4-minute video that describes baby bottle tooth decay (available in other languages)	Public Health Foundation WIC Program 583 Monterey Pass Rd. Monterey Park, CA 91754 (818)570–4149
BBTD: A Professional Guide A 12-minute video on prevention for caregivers and health professionals	Dental Health Foundation 4340 Redwood Hwy., #319 San Rafael, CA 94903 (415)499–4648
American Dental Association (1995) *Baby Bottle Tooth Decay Prevention* *Brushing Magic with Dudley and Dee* *Dudley in Nutrition Land* *Dudley Visits the Dentist* *Dudley's Classroom Adventure* *Flash That Smile* *The Haunted Mouth* *It's Dental Flossophy, Charlie Brown* *Toothbrushing with Charlie Brown*	American Dental Association 211 E. Chicago Ave. Chicago, IL 60611-2678 (800)947–4746 Fax: (312)440–3542

(continued)

Table A–2   Selected Dental Health Educational Resources (continued)

Item and Description	Source
Brochures	
Protect Your Child's Teeth	Dental Health Foundation (listed above)
Nutrition Education Materials	Dairy Council of Wisconsin Westmont, IL
Advice for Parents *Baby Bottle Tooth Decay* *Basic Brushing* *Basic Flossing* *Benefits of Sealants* *Diet and Tooth Decay* *Happiness Is a Healthy Smile* *Smokeless Tobacco* *Stages of Tooth Development* *Your Child's Teeth*	American Dental Association (listed above)
Posters	
Toothbrushing chart Flossing chart Baby bottle tooth decay Progress of tooth decay Smokeless tobacco Youth posters (variety)	American Dental Association (listed above)
Slides	
Today's Dentistry Everything you need for a community presentation	American Dental Association (listed above)
Books	

Growing Up Cavity Free by Stephen J.
    Moss, DDS; "A parents guide to
    prevention"
	Quintessence Publishing Co.
	551 N. Kimberly Dr.
	Carol Stream, IL 60188-1881
	(900)621–0387

The Bully Brothers Trick the Tooth Fairy
    by Mike Thaler 1993
Brush Your Teeth Please,
    by Joshua Morris
The Magic School Bus,
Inside Your Mouth (activity book) and
A Trip to the Water Works, by Linda Beech
The Very Hungry Caterpillar,
    by Eric Carle
Loose Tooth, by Steven Kroll
	Available in most bookstores or by
	    special order

Supplies	
Big tooth model Big toothbrush	ADA (listed above) also available at Block Drug Company 105 Academy Street Jersey City, NJ 07302 (800)365–6500
Anti-tobacco/smokeless tobacco brochures, posters, and books	American Cancer Society (800)4–CANCER
Bright Smiles/Bright Futures Grades 1 and 3 and preschool	Colgate One Colgate Way Canton, MA 02021 (800)334–7734

Table A–2   Selected Dental Health Educational Resources (continued)

Item and Description	Source
Tooth stickers, notepads, borders, posters, etc.	Carson-Dellrosa's P.O. Box 35665 Greensboro, NC 27425 (800)321–0943
Teacher supplies	Consult local phone book
Posters Video (Sparkel) Brochures Toothbrushes Toothpaste Dental health month Activity books Stickers Bookmarks	CREST Procter & Gamble Oral Health Products Professional Sales P.O. Box 148013 Fairfield, CA 45014-9923 (800)543–2577
Chairside aid Dental care kits Brochures Toothbrushes Toothpaste	Colgate Oral Pharmaceuticals One Colgate Way Canton, MA 02021 (800)225–3156
Floss Mouth rinse Fluoride Toothbrushes	Oral B Laboratories One Lagoon Dr. Redwood City, CA 94065 (800)446–7252
Toothpaste Floss/fluoride Fluoride Toothbrushes	Johnson & Johnson Dental Care Divison New Brunswick, NJ 08903 (800)526–3967
Floss ACT Toothbrushes/covers Fluoride Toothbrushing timers	Plak Smackers 4015 Indus Way Riverside, CA 92503 (800)558–6684 Fax: (909)734–4750
Disclosing tablets Gloves/masks Floss/Floss holder Kits Toothbrushes	E-Z Floss P.O. Box 2292 Palm Springs, CA 92263 CA: (800)227–0208 Nationwide: (800)458–6872

Recommended Dental Titles

Several books with a dental health focus can be recommended for use in the elementary school classroom. New titles are constantly being released, and the dental health educator should make an effort to review these resources periodically. Table A–3 presents an alphabetical list of several recommended titles.

Table A–3 Recommended Dental Titles

Title	Author	Price ($)	Publisher
Bear in the Hospital	Bucknall	11.95	Penguin
Alfred Goes to the Hospital	Schanzer	5.95	Barron's
All About Our Bodies Our Teeth	NL (author not listed)	4.50	Heian International
Anna's Special Present	Tsutsui	10.95	Penguin USA
Arthur's Tooth (hardcover)	Brown	14.95	Little, Brown
Arthur's Tooth (paperback)	Brown	4.95	Little, Brown
Arthur's Tooth (book and cassette)	Brown	7.95	Little, Brown
Arthur's Loose Tooth	Hoban	3.50	HarperCollins
B. Bears Go to the Doctor (puppet)	Berenstain	2.95	Random House
B. Bears Go to the Dentist	Berenstain	2.95	Random House
B. Bears Go to the Doctor	Berenstain	2.25	Random House
B. Bears Visit Dentist (book and cassette)	Berenstain	5.95	Random House
Bear's Toothache	McPhail	5.95	Little, Brown
Betsy and the Chicken	Wolde	4.95	Random House
Betsy and the Doctor	Wolde	4.95	Random House
Big Bird Goes to the Doctor	SESST	2.95	Western
Brush Your Teeth Please	NL	9.95	Random House
BSLS 43 Karen's Toothache	Martin	2.95	Scholastic Book Service
Dilly Goes to the Dentist	Bradman	9.95	Viking Penguin
Going to the Dentist	Borgardt	8.95	Simon & Schuster
Going to the Dentist	Civardi	3.95	EDC
Great Zopper Toothpaste Cyda	Boch	2.50	Bantam
Serpent's Tooth Mystery	Dixon	3.50	Simon & Schuster
Hospital Journal	Banks	7.95	Penguin USA
Hospital Story	Stein	8.95	Walker & Company
How Many Teeth?	Showers	4.95	HarperCollins
How the Tooth Fairy Got Her Job	Henry	3.95	Purple Turtle
Just Going to the Dentist	Mayer	2.25	Western
Little Rabbit's Loose Tooth	Bate	4.99	Random House
Loose Tooth (hardcover)	Kroll	13.95	Holiday House

(continued)

Table A–3   Recommended Dental Titles (continued)

Title	Author	Price ($)	Publisher
Loose Tooth (paperback)	Kroll	2.50	Scholastic Book Service
Maggie and the Emergency Room	NL	2.25	Random House
Martin and the Tooth Fairy 3	Chardiet-Maccarone	2.50	Scholastic Book Service
Missing Tooth	Cole	3.50	Random House
Mr. Rogers Going to the Dentist	Rodgers	5.95	Putnam's
My Dentist	Rockwell	3.95	Wm. Morrow
My Tooth Is Loose	Silverman	3.50	Penguin USA
Rita Goes to the Hospital	NL	2.25	Random House
Rosie's Baby Tooth	MacDonald	12.95	MacMillan/Atheneum
Ruth's Loose Tooth	NL	5.95	Price, Stern, Sloan
Saber Toothed Cat	NL	5.95	Simon & Schuster
Serpent's Tooth	Paxson	4.99	Avon Books
Teeth	NL	3.95	Steck-Vaughn/Raintree
Tooth Book	Lesieg	6.95	Random House
Tooth Fairy	Wood	3.95	Child's Play International
Tooth Fairy Book	Kovacs	9.95	Running Press
Tooth Gnasher Superflash	Pinkwater	3.95	Macmillan/Atheneum
Tooth Witch (hardcover)	Karlin	11.95	Harper & Row
Tooth Witch (paperback)	Karlin	4.95	HarperCollins
Toothpaste Millionaire	Merrill	4.95	Houghton Mifflin
Trip to the Dentist	Linn	9.95	HarperCollins
When I See My Dentist	Kuklin	13.95	Macmillan
Who Put That Hair In My Toothbrush?	Spinelli	3.50	Dell
Why Am I Going to the Hospital?	Ciliotta	12.00	Carol

NL = author not listed.

gloſſary

Abscess A collection of pus in the tissues, usually due to infection by bacteria.

Acid A compound having a sour taste and the ability to turn litmus paper red and destroy enamel.

Alveolar bone The bone in which the teeth are embedded.

Amalgam An alloy, composed mainly of silver, tin, and mercury, used for filling teeth.

Anterior teeth The central and lateral incisors and the cuspids of either jaw.

Arch, dental The horseshoe-shaped bony ridge in which the teeth are embedded.

Bacteria (germ) A large group of typically one-celled microorganisms, many of which are disease-producing.

Bicuspid (premolar) The first and second biscuspids are found just in back of each cuspid. These teeth have two cusps (points) and are used to tear and grind food.

Bruxism Clenching or grinding of the teeth, usually during sleep.

Calculus Hardened plaque that forms and adheres to the crowns and roots of the teeth; also called tarter.

Canine tooth See *cuspid.*

Caries A localized bacterial disease process that destroys tooth structure and produces a cavity.

Cavity The decayed portion of a tooth.

Cementum A calcified tissue that forms the outer layer of the roots of the teeth.

Crown The portion of a tooth that is covered with enamel and is visible in the mouth above the gum line.

Cuspid (canine) A sharp-pointed tooth located between the first bicuspid and the lateral incisor used for tearing food, sometimes called eye tooth.

Decalcify To remove calcium salts from the bone or teeth by biochemical action.

Decay To become impaired or rotted, as a cavity.

Deciduous teeth (primary) Those teeth that are shed at a certain age; baby teeth.

Dental hygienist A professionally educated person qualified and licensed to provide certain specified dental services such as cleaning the teeth (prophylaxis) and educating the public in good dental health practices.

Dentifrice (toothpaste or toothpowder) A cleaning substance for the teeth.

Dentin The hard, dense, calcified tissue that forms the body of the tooth underneath the enamel and cementum.

Dentures A set of artificial teeth.

Enamel The smooth, hard, outer layer of the tooth crown.

Eruption The process of teeth breaking through the gums, as "cutting" teeth.

Extraction Removing or pulling a tooth.

Filling A material (usually gold, silver, plastic, or cement or similar materials) inserted in a prepared cavity in a tooth.

Fissure A fault in the surface of a tooth caused by imperfect enamel formation.

Fluoridation The adjustment of the fluoride content in the public water supply to prevent or reduce tooth decay.

Fluoride A compound of fluorine and another element.

> **Topical fluoride** Application of fluoride to the teeth for decay prevention.

Gingiva (gums) The tissue that covers the alveolar bone of the upper and lower jaws and surrounds the necks of the teeth.

Gingivitis Inflammation involving the gums and gingival tissues.

Gumboil (abscess) An inflamed and painful part of the gum tissue caused by an abscessed or diseased tooth.

Hygiene, oral Cleanliness or proper care of the mouth and teeth.

Impacted tooth A tooth that is embedded in the alveolar bone in such a way that its eruption is prevented.

Incisors Any one of the four front teeth of the upper or lower jaw.

    Central incisors The two front teeth in both the upper and lower jaws.

    Lateral incisors The teeth that are situated on either side of the central incisors in both the upper and lower jaws.

Malocclusion An irregularity of tooth position and poor fitting together of the teeth when the jaws are closed.

Mandible The lower jawbone.

Mastication The act of chewing.

Maxilla The upper jawbone.

Molar A tooth used for grinding; a back tooth of which there are usually three on each side of both jaws.

Neck of tooth The area of the tooth that forms the junction of the crown and root.

Nerve of tooth The nerve fiber found in the pulp, which supplies the tooth with feeling.

Orthodontic appliance A device used by an orthodontist to guide teeth into proper position.

Orthodontics The specialty that deals with the prevention and correction of malocclusion.

Partial denture An appliance that replaces one or more missing teeth.

Periodontal membrane A layer of tissue made up of tiny fibers that help hold the tooth in its socket.

Periodontitis (pyorrhea) Inflammation of the supporting tissues of the teeth, usually resulting in a discharge of pus, foul odor, and possible looseness of the teeth.

Permanent teeth The second set of teeth (32 in number); those that follow the primary teeth.

Pit A small indentation in the crown of a tooth.

Plaque A thin, tenacious, sticky, film-like deposit—made up of a protein substance and microorganisms—that adheres to the tooth.

Prophylaxis The professional cleaning of teeth by a dentist or dental hygienist to aid in the prevention of dental disease.

Prosthetic appliance An artificial replacement for missing teeth and other oral tissues (see also *dentures*).

Protrusion Projection of the upper front teeth often caused by thumbsucking; a form of malocclusion.

Pulp chamber The chamber in the core area of the tooth that is filled with blood vessels, nerves, and connective tissues.

Root The part of the tooth that is normally beneath the gums and anchors the tooth in the jawbone.

Root canal The passageway in the root through which blood vessels and nerves enter the pulp chamber.

Saliva The clear, alkaline secretion from the glands discharging into the mouth.

Sodium fluoride A chemical combination of sodium and fluorine.

Space maintainer An appliance inserted in place of a missing tooth to prevent the other teeth from drifting.

Stannous fluoride A chemical combination of tin and fluorine.

Tarter Hardened plaque that forms and adheres to the crowns and roots of the teeth.

Temporomandibular joint The hinge of the jaw just in front of each ear on which the mandible or lower jaw swings.

Vincent's infection A disease that attacks the gums and other parts of the mouth and throat; also known as trench mouth.

Wisdom tooth The third or last molar in each jaw.

X-rays A technique to show detailed images of structures that are not ordinarily visible.

biblioqraphy

American Dental Association. (1980). *Learning about your oral health: A prevention-oriented school program* (Vols. 1–4). Chicago: Author.

American Society of Dentistry for Children. (1975) *Tooth talk. A teacher's guide flip chart K–3.* Chicago IL: Author.

Bowen, P.L. (1994). Teaching oral health in the classroom. *Dental Teamwork,* January–February, 26–27.

Brown, W. (1995). *Facts on water fluoridation.* Sacramento, CA: California Department of Health Services.

Children's Dental Disease Prevention Program, S.B. 111, Health and Safety Code §§ 360–375.5 (1979). Article 4.5 Children's Dental Disease Prevention Program.

Dembo, Myron H. (1994). *Applying Educational Psychology,* 5th ed. Longman Publishing Group.

Hunter, M.C. *The Teaching Process,_____.*

The Family School Partnership Act, AB2590 (1995, State of California).

Merriam-Webster's collegiate dictionary (10th ed.). (1993). Springfield, MA: Merriam-Webster.

Moss, S.J. (1993). *Growing up cavity free.* Chicago: Quintessence Publishing.

Renner, G. (1985). *The instructor's survival kit.* PFR Training Associates Limited.

U.S. Department of Health and Human Services, Public Health Service. (1991). *Healthy people 2000. National health promotion and disease prevention objectives.* Washington, DC: Author.

Yee, H. (1982). *Mini activity packet for teachers. State dental disease prevention program.* Sacramento: State Dept of CA.

Other Related Titles

**Dental Assistant
Program Review and Exam
Preparation (PREP)**
Andujo
1997, ISBN 0-8385-1513-4, A1513-9

**Appleton & Lange's Quick
Review
Dental Assistant**
Andujo
1998, ISBN 0-8385-1526-6, A1526-1

**Appleton & Lange's Review of
Dental Hygiene**
Fourth Edition
Barnes & Waring
1995, ISBN 0-8385-0230-X, A0230-1

Primary Preventive Dentistry
Fifth Edition
Harris & Garcia-Godoy
December 1998, ISBN 0-8385-8129-3,
A8129-7

**Essentials of Dental Radiography
For Dental Assistants and
Hygienists**
Sixth Edition
Johnson et al.
October 1998, ISBN 0-8385-2222-X,
A2222-6

**Dental Anatomy
A Self-Instructional Program**
Tenth Edition
Karst & Smith
1998, ISBN 0-8385-1492-8, A1492-6

Peridontal Instrumentation
Second Edition
Pattison & Pattison
1992, ISBN 0-8385-7804-7, A7804-6

**Head & Neck Histology &
Anatomy
A Self-Instructional Program**
Smith & Karst
January 1999, ISBN 0-8385-3652-2,
A3652-3

To order or for more information, visit your local health science bookstore
or call Appleton & Lange toll free at **1-800-423-1359.**